Awareness

C000066713

Awareness: What it is, What it does is an accessible up-to-date summary of scientific thinking about the nature of consciousness. Relevant, basic facts about the brain and the physical world are described including what is understood about time in these contexts. Chris Nunn then examines in detail various theories of consciousness highlighting their strengths and weaknesses and comparing quantum and neural theories. Some implications of these new ideas, particularly those with consequences for medicine and psychiatry, are also discussed.

The study of awareness is currently a fast developing and controversial area. This book sets out in a manner intended to be easily read many of the most exciting theoretical and experimental advances. It will be of interest to a wide range of academics, professionals and students.

Chris Nunn is a former Consultant Psychiatrist, based in Southampton. He combined his role providing services for local communities with extensive research interests in mind/body relationships and awareness.

Awareness

What it is, What it does

Chris Nunn

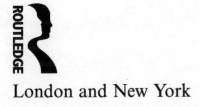

London and New York

First published 1996
by Routledge
11 New Fetter Lane, London EC4P 4EE

Simultaneously published in the USA and Canada
by Routledge
29 West 35th Street, New York, NY 10001

Typeset in Times by Routledge
Printed and bound in Great Britain by
TJ Press (Padstow) Ltd., Cornwall

British Library Cataloguing in Publication Data
A catalogue record for this book is available from the British Library

Library of Congress Cataloguing in Publication Data
A catalogue record for this book has been requested

ISBN 0–415–13226–6 (hbk)
ISBN 0–415–13227–4 (pbk)

Contents

Acknowledgements

I am indebted to all the writers mentioned in this book, but would like to single out Roger Penrose whose *Emperor's New Mind*, published in 1989, first brought to my attention many of the ideas discussed here. Reading him was better than changing into something comfortable after a day wearing shoes that pinched and a collar that was too tight, but felt similar.

I also owe much to the 'consciousness group' here in Southampton. Its leading lights are Chris Clarke, a mathematician who is now dean of the faculty, and Doug Newman, professor of physics. Chris has done his best to educate me in the use of the many rather esoteric concepts needed to get to grips with awareness. My failings are my fault, not his. Doug has followed his own valuable line of thought concerning neural nets and the role of self-models in generating consciousness. His book on this is due out soon. It is of great interest, and the fact that I do not agree with all of it has helped me to overcome natural laziness and sort out my own ideas. He has also been so kind as to review sections of my manuscript with appropriate scepticism.

Others who have provided most helpful criticisms of the manuscript are my son Miles and my colleague Brian Barraclough. Many thanks to them, too. A particularly beneficent influence has been that of Ian Marshall, both through the work that he has published with Danah Zohar, his wife, and especially in the course of an always stimulating and often enlightening correspondence.

That I have had the time to write is thanks to the support of my wife, Ruth, and the skill of my surgeon Frank McGinn.

It's a pity that there is no more appropriate pronoun to use than 'my' in relation to other people. This should not be taken to imply possession of any sort but is simply a means of referring to those who, from the goodness of their hearts, have taken an interest in me or in this book.

The author would like to thank the following for permission to reproduce short extracts: J. W. Brown from 'Psychology of Time Awareness', *Brain and Cognition* (1990: 14, 144–64), courtesy of Academic Press, Florida; F. Crick and C. Koch from 'The Problem of Consciousness' (1992), courtesy of Scientific American, New York; D. W. DeMott from *Toposcopic Studies of Learning* (1970), courtesy of Charles C. Thomas, Publisher, Springfield, Illinois; G. Dougary from 'Between the Lines', *Times Magazine* (5 March 1994); T. Honderich from *Mindwaves* (edited by Blakemore and Greenfield) (1987), courtesy of Basil Blackwell, Oxford; A. J. Marcel from 'Conscious and Unconscious Perception', *Cognitive Psychology* (1983: 15, 238–300), courtesy of Academic Press, Florida; J. S. Nicolis and I. Tsuda from 'Chaotic Dynamics of Information Processing', *Bulletin of Mathematical Biology* (1985: 47(3), 343–65), with the kind permission of Elsevier Science Ltd, Oxford; M. O'Donnell from 'Anecdotal Evidence: Persecuted by Counsellors', *Healthcare Management* (1994); R. Penrose, from *The Emperor's New Mind* (1989) by permission of Oxford University Press.

Every effort has been made to contact owners of copyright material which is reproduced in this book. In the event of a copyright query please contact the publishers.

Introduction

This book is about consciousness, though I prefer to use the term 'awareness' instead. Consciousness can imply self-awareness and, for a philosopher, may carry overtones of intentionality, emotionality or whatever. I've written mainly about the basic phenomenon that underlies everyday experience and lights up, so to speak, things like my idea of myself, my feelings at this moment and so forth. Although people have some sense of 'I' almost constantly present either somewhere in the background or, more often, well to the forefront of their consciousness, the pure awareness described by Zen masters and very occasionally experienced by many people does exist. All sense of person and other common attributes of consciousness are lost when in such a state, but awareness remains.

There are philosophers and others who claim that it is wrong to suppose that awareness can be meaningfully discussed independently of some particular set of attributes which they happen to favour, but most of their arguments are too involved to concern us here. Some end up asserting that conscious experience is a sort of illusion which does not really occur in the way that we experience it (e.g. Dennett, 1991). Quite a lot of ingenuity is needed to reach seemingly ridiculous conclusions of this type! All the same it has to be admitted that intentionality, which simply means that consciousness is always about something, probably is inseparable from awareness even if the content in question may very occasionally be nothing other than awareness of being aware. Moreover, there is experimental evidence of illusory aspects to what we experience, especially in connection with the apparent timing of awareness. However, I've avoided direct philosophical discussion of issues of this sort as the arguments involved tend to be lengthy, often circular and usually inconclusive. The approach taken here is to assume that awareness is the basic phenomenon and to look at what might generate and accompany it.

The book grew out of some research on the nature of consciousness that I did recently. Talking about the research to colleagues brought the surprising realisation that some of them could not really see the point of it, though we were all working with the mentally ill and awareness forms the basis of mentality, including sick mentality. It had seemed to me obvious that getting some idea of what consciousness really is would be nice from a professional point of view, as well as satisfying to ordinary curiosity. Many of those colleagues who did share my curiosity had themselves dismissed the problem years ago as too difficult for serious consideration. On the whole, medical and nursing students to whom I spoke were less daunted by the difficulties and more ready to think about the issues involved than were trained staff. In fact the whole field of consciousness studies is opening up fast. Although by no means straightforward, it may not turn out to be inherently much more difficult than, say, molecular biology. Agreed it's more mysterious than molecular biology at present, though no more strange to us now than was the concept of Life to a nineteenth-century biochemist, but that may be partly because so many have thought it unapproachable.

It therefore seemed a good idea to try to get the whole range of concepts needed for approaching an understanding of awareness into one brief book. Busy people would be unlikely to read anything too long. Because of brevity this account is quite superficial in places but not, I hope, misleading. There's a bias towards a particular view of the basis of awareness, but this is clearly signposted in the text, and my own guess is that it will eventually turn out to have been correct; also, having a definite bias helps the story-line along. Quite a range of books espousing particular, individual views about consciousness have been published recently (*The Astonishing Hypothesis* by Francis Crick got the most publicity, though the title is something of a misnomer when applied to the view that he favours). I don't know of any attempt other than mine to tackle nearly the full range of ideas, excluding only the purely philosophical ones, currently involved in consciousness studies.

A batch of excellent, if lengthy, works on the subject appeared in 1989. They were by Edelman, Lockwood and Penrose. Lockwood's book, although in some ways the most thoughtful of the three, did not attract an extensive readership, but those by Edelman and Penrose provoked a great deal of interest and defined two opposed ways of looking at the basis of awareness. A lot of people have been working on the implications and applications of these two approaches over the last six years, so it's now possible to add to, as well as summarise, what they wrote. Penrose's own follow-up, to be called *Shadows of the Mind*, is in press as I'm typing this.

The plan followed here is to outline in the first two Chapters basic facts and findings about the brain, and about how it works in relation to awareness. Parts of Chapter 1 in particular could prove tedious to readers who already have the relevant background knowledge; skimming is recommended in that event, and is facilitated by the sub-headings. Then, because the Penrose-type approach to consciousness depends on quantum theory, an account of relevant aspects of this is given in Chapter 3 for those unfamiliar with it. If the account is hard to understand, I hope kind readers will attribute any problems to the notorious difficulty of the theory rather than to my incompetence! The concepts involved are fascinating, and I hope to have conveyed some of that fascination. Next, various theories concerning consciousness itself are described in Chapter 4. After a nostalgic look at the old idea that awareness is an attribute of the separate soul possessed by each of us, it is pointed out that there are at present only two scientifically valid ways of regarding consciousness; the first is to think of it as a direct consequence of patterns of neural activity of the sort that have been familiar to brain scientists since the time of Sherrington early in this century (depolarisation waves, neurotransmitter release, etc.), which emerges when such patterns become sufficiently elaborate; the alternative, second view regards awareness as a phenomenon based on properties of the brain that can be understood only in terms of quantum theory.

The rest of the book is occupied by looking at the evidence (Chapter 5) or some of the more general considerations (Chapters 6 and 8) that might lead to a preference for one or other of the basic approaches to awareness. Chapters 6,7 and 8 also deal with some of the implications of the theories, particularly the quantum-based ones. It turns out that the consequences for medicine, if a Penrose-type approach to awareness should eventually prove valid, would be of considerable practical importance (Chapter 8). Finally, Chapter 9 is a brief speculation on the theme that a quantum view of consciousness might allow resurrection of something very similar to the old idea of a soul having 'thing-like' properties.

That's the intention, but there are obstacles to achieving it in a satisfactory manner on top of problems caused by contemporary ignorance about relevant facts. One such difficulty arises because it's necessary to cover a field ranging from the mathematical basis of quantum theory, through neurology and psychology to things like art appreciation. Thus it's impossible to get the descriptive level right for everyone all of the time. Depending on your own specialised knowledge, kind reader, you are likely to find my account ridiculously basic in some places and quite abstruse in others. If bored, skim; if, on the other hand, you get into difficulties please refer to the glossary which may help. If that's no good, I suggest skipping to the section headed 'Conclusions' (one is to be found at the end of each chapter, except Chapter 9) which sums up the narrative and arguments, allowing people to go on to the next chapter without missing anything essential.

While on the subject of a glossary, I must confess to a thoroughly idiosyncratic use of the word 'quale' (plural 'qualia'). This is normally defined as a perceptual quality such as redness, or blueness, or the experience of hearing middle C played on a piano. However, such experiences are almost always inseparably tied up with a whole rag-bag of associates, for example other visual impressions, feelings of various sorts, awarenesses of meanings, knowledge that there is an ache in your big toe and that you are having this ache, etc., etc. I therefore use 'quale' to refer, not to isolated perceptual qualities, but as convenient shorthand for the content, however complex it may be, of any moment of experience. What a 'moment' might be is discussed in Chapter 2.

The next obstacle is even more basic, and is due to the fact that a quale is directly accessible only to the person having it. If he or she is to report on it, it must be remembered. The same problem arises for the individual, introspective person because, if one is to be aware that one has had an awareness, one has to remember it. To get side-tracked into philosophy for a few seconds, the phrase 'aware that one has had an awareness' may raise fears of an infinite regress but these would not be justified as the first 'aware' is definitely dependent on memory whereas the second 'awareness' may not involve memory at all and, even if it does, is in a different relationship to memory from the first.

What this boils down to is that one can never be sure of what might constitute the full range of awareness. Some people believe that memory plays an essential role in generating consciousness, but if they are wrong there are likely to be whole areas of awareness that escape our knowledge because they don't get into memory. The cerebellum (see glossary if necessary), for example, is often thought to be an unconscious neural servo-mechanism, but perhaps activity in it is not directly incorporated in reported awareness because it lacks the necessary memory mechanisms. There's already new evidence (Kim *et al.*, 1994) that, contrary to earlier views about its functions, it is involved in cognitive processes associated with awareness. From the opposite point of view, the hippocampus, which is known to have an important role in memory, has been regarded by some as a potential seat of consciousness. It's equally probable, however, that the evidence for this is due solely to awareness being more likely to get remembered when occurring in an area that specialises in memory.

Because of this limitation, we can talk about where awareness *is*, but are on very unsure ground if we try to talk about where it *isn't*; something which causes difficulties for both theorists and experimentalists that will only be overcome when a good, objective test for the occurrence of consciousness is developed. What's needed is the machine that allowed Mr Spock of *Star Trek* to report, 'There are two life-forms down there, Jim'. As will emerge in due course, there's a real possibility that a device like this might exist one day.

To round off this introduction, I can't resist re-quoting here the Chinese saying that Lockwood (1989) used to set the theme for his book:

We are that in which the earth comes to appreciate itself.

Provided that the earth is regarded as including the body in which 'we' reside, this gives the neatest possible one-line summary of the human condition. We *are* our experience which consists of reflecting the world in the magic mirror of awareness. Anything else that we might regard as constituting 'us' is unconscious and so has only indirect reality for us.

REFERENCES

Dennett, D.C. (1991) *Consciousness Explained*, Penguin Books: Harmondsworth.

Edelman, G.M. (1989) *The Remembered Present: A Biological Theory of Consciousness*, Basic Books: New York.

Kim, S-G., Ugurbil K. and Strick, P.L. (1994) 'Activation of a Cerebellar Output Nucleus During Cognitive Processing', *Science* 265, 949–51.

Lockwood, M. (1989) *Mind, Brain and the Quantum: The Compound 'I'*, Basil Blackwell: Oxford.

Penrose, R. (1989) *The Emperor's New Mind*, Oxford University Press: Oxford.

1 The boundaries of awareness

It seems quite a good idea to approach an understanding of awareness by first delimiting the sort of space that it occupies. You can get a surprisingly accurate impression of what an unknown animal will look like by seeing where it lives, what it eats and so forth. The same strategy may work in relation to awareness, though most writers, especially if they are philosophers, take the opposite approach. They often try to define a whole collection of what they regard as essential attributes of consciousness, things like intentionality, self-reference, emotional tone (the list varies from writer to writer), and then imagine what sort of space would be filled by their particular animal.

It is not so easy, of course, to know which boundaries may be most usefully explored. Looking to see if something builds nests will not tell you if it is a bird or a squirrel – you would need to examine the nest lining or the remains of its food for that. As far as awareness is concerned there are a few very obvious limitations, so obvious that they are often taken for granted. For instance, you cannot have awareness without a brain to have it in, or at least to provide an origin for it if 'out of the body' experiences can be taken at face value (there is ongoing debate about whether they are an illusion produced by dying or highly-stressed brains, or whether they are veridical). The brain has to be in reasonably good physical shape and needs to use a lot of energy if it is to remain aware. However, damage to some areas will not greatly affect awareness whereas damage to other sometimes quite small bits, particularly if they are in the brain stem, will totally abolish sentience. Awareness can be abolished almost equally well by flooding the brain with small fat-soluble molecules such as ether or halothane (a popular anaesthetic), which do not necessarily reduce energy consumption much.

Why anaesthetics work is an important mystery which will presumably be solved only when we know what awareness really is.

The evidence so far (Franks and Lieb, 1994) suggests that they abolish consciousness by causing small changes of shape in various protein constituents of nerve cells. On current theories of brain function one might predict that the relevant proteins would be those comprising receptors in nerve cell membranes, but in fact it seems unlikely that effects on these are primarily responsible for anaesthesia because receptors are mostly resistant to the concentrations of anaesthetics that are used clinically. Where they act remains unknown.

In brief, what we are hunting is clearly a product of some of the more energetic sorts of brain activity, but probably not all of them. It might even be regarded as a surprisingly robust product because quite gross interference is needed to abolish it for more than a few moments. The most important thing to focus on here may be the high energy demands made by sentience. In humans, as much as 30 per cent of the body's resting energy expenditure is due to the brain which accounts for around 3 per cent of one's weight. This is very costly in Darwinian terms and suggests that awareness must carry some overwhelming evolutionary advantage, or at least must be inseparably associated with some such advantage. It will be worth remembering this later on when we shall find reasons for thinking that consciousness might be nothing more than an irrelevant epiphenomenon of brain activity. The energy costs of awareness are not proof that consciousness does useful things, but are a strong indication that it may.

So far, we have identified an animal which lives in the brain and may, just conceivably, occasionally emerge beyond its lair. To get a better picture of it, we shall have to examine its habitat more closely and from a whole lot of different angles. This Chapter will start off dealing with the more 'spatial' aspects of its environment and then go on to look at some of its behaviour; the next chapter concerns the time-related side of things.

THE NEURAL SUBSTRATE

The brain has some ten billion nerve cells and an even larger number of supporting cells which are thought to do things like provide the nerve cells with nutrition and maintain the insulating sheaths round nerve fibres. They are not generally thought to play any direct part in the work of the brain, though this is not known for certain. They could well, for instance, have a primary role in learning and memory by pruning unnecessary nerve cell connections or by killing off unwanted cells. It has even been semi-seriously proposed (Rowlands, 1983) that the supporting cells form the basis of a 'second' nervous system operating at far higher frequencies than the primary system made up of neurones. There is recent direct evidence (Nedergaard, 1994) that stimulating astrocytes, which are one of the varieties of supporting cell, can modulate the activity of neighbouring neurones. All the same, it is usually assumed that the seat of awareness is in the nerve cells themselves or some functional aspect of their interconnections.

Nerve cells are unusual in several respects; once mature, they cannot divide and many of them live as long as their owner; they have immensely long processes which often branch like a tree; cell to cell influences are far more elaborate and precise than is the case for most types of cell. Nerve cell processes typically extend over a few millimetres but may sometimes reach a metre or more. Each cell may be in touch with as many as ten thousand others. They communicate via specific chemicals (neurotransmitters) released by one cell which activate receptors on another. Some of these chemicals are precisely targeted in places where the processes of one cell are almost touching another, but others are released into the fluid bathing the brain or into the bloodstream and so reach their targets that way. There are a lot (certainly over 50 distinct chemicals) of different neurotransmitters, and some of them are known to influence more than one type of receptor. The whole set-up is, in other words, inordinately complicated.

The internal structure of nerve cells, like that of cells in general, is highly ordered. There is a so-called cytoskeleton (i.e. cellular skeleton) which extends internally to the furthest ramification of each nerve cell. It is made of microtubules; miniature tube-like structures composed of a variety of different, though related, proteins whch are given the generic name of tubulin. These microtubules are hollow with an internal diameter of 25 nanometers and themselves have an ordered, regular structure (a skewed hexagonal lattice – see Del Giudice *et al.*, 1986). Apart from maintaining cell shape, they are thought also to have a role in transporting chemicals within cells and in governing some of their functions.

One can try to get an understanding of the brain in three basic ways and a whole lot of more fancy ones. The basic approaches are via anatomy, electrical activity or chemical sub-typing. There is a problem here because of the vast amount of information that exists about each of the basic approaches and the reams of speculation concerning the fancy ones. It would be only too easy to bore any reader to tears with detail, so all that will be given is an impressionistic outline of the most important features of each approach. Anyone wanting more solid fare will need to refer to the voluminous technical literature.

ANATOMY

The two most striking characteristics of the brain are that its largest component (the cerebral cortex) is essentially two-dimensional (2D) and that, despite its rather porridge-like external appearance, the whole thing has a very complicated but highly-ordered structure. Both of these features must have implications for an understanding of awareness, even if it's not too clear what the implications are.

The cortex consists of a six-layered sheet of cells that is much rumpled and folded in humans but in rabbits, for instance, is quite smooth. This two-dimensionality seems natural in relation to the visual cortex which can be regarded as a complex reflection of the two-dimensional surface of the retina of the eye. However, it already appears dysfunctional in relation to the motor cortex which maps movements occurring in three-dimensional (3D) space, while intellectual and emotional functions would require a multi-dimensional space to be represented economically. It is a considerable handicap, one would suppose, to be confined to 2D for handling higher functions.

The sheet-like structure of the cortex is an ideal medium on which to draw maps of the environment, and the evidence suggests that this is just what often happens, though why it should be a good thing to create sketches of one's surroundings in this way is another matter. Columns of cortical cells representing, for example, contours or splashes of colour perceived by the retina or tones distinguished by the cochlea of the ear are so positioned as to form a map or diagram of these features of the environment. There is evidence (Skarda and Freeman, 1987) that even smells are distinguished by their different spatial representations in the olfactory bulb of rabbits.

All the same, it should not be supposed that the sensory cortex is even remotely like a photographic film served by 'cameras' that can pick up sound, touch and smell as well as light. This is illustrated by the fact that the parts of the visual cortex analysing colour, contour and movement are quite widely separated from one another, and similar considerations probably apply to other cortical areas. It is altogether remarkable that we should perceive a cricket ball as a red round thing flying through the air, instead of as an area of redness – and a round entity – and a movement. The so-called 'binding problem' (why awareness should appear unified) occurs even at basic perceptual levels like this and the sheet-like structure of the cortex makes it all the more of a puzzle. There is no little man inside the brain, and no master neurone to look at all the separate diagrams and integrate them. How then do the contours of a caricature, say, perceived by the occipital cortex and the emotional reaction to it, which is probably represented in the frontal lobes some 10 centimetres away, both combine to form one quale? This question is probably central to reaching an understanding of awareness, and is one to which we shall keep returning.

Another feature of these cortical sheets has become so familiar that it rarely causes wonder. This is that the left hand deals with the right side of the body and the world, and vice versa. There are all sorts of wiring complications as a result. For instance, fibres from the half of each eye farthest from the nose go to the same side of the brain while those from the half nearer to the nose go to the opposite side of the brain (if you think about it for a moment, you will see that this is so that the right side of the brain can deal with the left half of visual space and vice versa). Of course functions without a spatial location do not have to be treated in this way and language, for example, is usually mainly a left hemisphere function. It is often said that the left hemisphere specialises in sequential, logical analysis while the right hemisphere deals in intuitive *Gestalts*. There is some truth in this but it could as well be a consequence as a cause of the fact that language, a quintessentially sequential function, sited itself on the left. But why should functions with a spatial component be located as they are? It looks as if the cortex is in truth a mirror of the world, albeit a highly selective and very distorting one.

The basic design is so odd, and apparently inefficient, that it must be signalling the existence of some design constraint or constraints of which we are ignorant. A very interesting suggestion made as long ago as 1970 by DeMott may be relevant here. He thought that the cortex can be regarded as a series of two-dimensional arrays of feature detectors and that sequences of *patterns* of activity in these underlie recognition, recall and the prediction of future events at all levels of sophistication from the prediction of the outcome of contracting a muscle to predicting what a friend will say next. It is certainly a most plausible idea, and one which for many years received far less attention than it deserved, though it has recently been resurrected in a slightly different form by Edelman (1989) who has produced strong arguments for the importance of 're-entrant' patterns of activity involving neuronal groups. If correct, or even approximately right, it may well be that a 2D structure is the only possible one for a large brain as the number of interconnections needed to transmit information from array to array might be impossibly large in 3D.

Further oddities abound in sub-cortical anatomy. The brain stem contains many, fairly distinct groups of nerve cells. Some of these are relay stations for nerve tracts on their way to or from the cortex, others are concerned with housekeeping functions such as breathing or temperature control, but some appear to play an essential, even a controlling, role underpinning cortical functions.

The attention of researchers has tended to wander from one such group of cells to another as time has passed. In the 1950s, the reticular activating system was the focus of interest which later wandered up to the thalamus. People are now tending to focus on smaller, more esoteric areas such as the locus coerulus. The latter contains only around 10,000 neurones (i.e. about a millionth of the total number), but sends connections to the whole of the rest of the nervous system from spinal chord to cortex. It may play a part in enhancing cognition (Berridge *et al.*, 1993). To researchers in the 1950s, the reticular activating system had appeared to play an even more central role, and was at one time regarded as a possible seat of consciousness.

DeMott (1970: 222) pointed out:

> The fact is, of course, that one can find connections between any two randomly selected points in the central nervous system, given enough patience and a goodly research grant. The conceptual difficulty with such systems is not that they imply connections which are not real, but that they encourage us to think of a certain group of structures as though they could, in any meaningful sense, be separated from the whole.

There's a lot of truth in this, but all the same the anatomically fairly-well-defined limbic system, for instance, does have a special role in short-term memory and flight/fight emotions. There are fairly localised areas controlling sleep/wakefulness and less well-localised ones dealing with pleasure/pain. There are, in other words, a whole range of specialised machines in the brain involving parts or all of the cortex and separate nuclei in the brain stem. The activities of these machines greatly influence the content of awareness and some of them may be necessary for any awareness to occur.

ELECTRICAL ACTIVITY

All cells maintain an electrical potential across their boundary membranes because they actively pump out a positive ion (sodium). Most of them are probably sensitive to applied electric fields which can, for example, affect the healing of wounds or the mobility of scavenging cells. Internal voltages between different parts of a single cell may also be important to functions like cell division. Neurones, of course, use this property of all cells in a highly specialised way in order to manipulate and transmit information.

If one bit of a nerve cell's membrane suffers a sufficient reduction in the voltage across it (called 'depolarisation'), neighbouring bits will follow suit so causing a wave of depolarisation to spread over the entire cell to its furthest branches. This can happen as a result of an applied electric current, but happens in nature when channels open in the membrane to allow positive ions to re-enter the cell. These channels are controlled by receptors which in turn are influenced by neurotransmitter chemicals. Some receptors, when stimulated by the right chemical, cause the channels to open while others cause them to close more firmly. Whether a wave of depolarisation will be triggered normally depends on a shifting balance of activity in stimulatory and inhibitory receptors. When a wave reaches the nerve terminal it triggers the release of some transmitter chemical that in turn influences the next cell. One can see intuitively how this system could be used to construct logic devices, though far more complex ones than the simple 'and', 'or', etc. devices to be found in computers, and it is, of course, a major focus of interest for neuroscientists and neural network specialists.

Depolarisation waves are transient (around 200/second is the peak rate at which they can occur) and spread quite slowly along nerve cell processes. The rate of spread is proportional to the diameter of the process. Where you need fast signalling, as a squid does from its brain to the muscles of its jet propulsion mechanism, one solution is to have huge axons. Those of the squid are a millimetre in diameter. What vertebrates, including humans, do instead is to insulate most longer processes, leaving the occasional gap. The wave then jumps from gap to gap, so travelling far faster than it otherwise would.

There are two other electrical phenomena worth a mention. One is that the depolarisation waves power small longitudinal currents along the length of axons. The magnetic component of these currents can be detected from outside the head, without even touching it, by the technique called magneto-encephalography (MEG). The other phenomenon is that areas where nerve processes are interwoven to form a sort of mat can undergo prolonged voltage changes, detectable by electrodes placed on the scalp, which can last far longer than individual depolarisation waves. Voltage changes associated with learning that endure for several days have been reported. Electro-encephalography (EEG; recording from electrodes placed on the scalp) picks up a combination of changes of this sort plus net current flows in the fluid surrounding groups of axons. The EEG in particular will keep turning up (like a good penny?) in all sorts of contexts throughout this book.

CHEMISTRY

Generally, the chemistry of nerve cells seems little different from that of other cells. They are more protected from the environment than most as there is a selective barrier between them and their blood supply which prevents many blood constituents from reaching them. Like all cells they use the hydrolysis of a molecule called ATP (and its very similar analogue GTP) as a fuel to power all that they do: however, nerve cells can use only glucose to create ATP, whereas most cells can also employ fats and proteins for this purpose. There may be interesting problems concerning how long thin nerve processes are maintained and supplied with enough energy, but these have not been clearly defined. Interest has tended to centre, therefore, on the variety of neurotransmitter chemicals.

Oddly enough, most is known about three of the rarer neurotransmitters. The more common ones, e.g. acetylcholine, glycine, GABA, have attracted less research over most of the last 40 years than the so-called monoamines (dopamine, noradrenaline 5-hydroxytryptamine, otherwise known as serotonin). This is because the monoamines seem to play a central part in mental illness. It is presumably more than coincidence that many of the neurones producing them have their cell bodies in the brain stem, although terminals releasing the monoamines are distributed over the whole of the nervous system as well as locally in the brain stem.

Like the brain stem/cortical 'machines' mentioned earlier, these chemicals appear to play semi-specific roles. Dopamine is involved in the maintenance of attention, while dopamine-blocking drugs tend to prevent hallucinations as well as causing muscle stiffness and tremor. Noradrenaline plays some rather ill-defined part in emotion and is probably the most important transmitter used by the locus coerulus in its role as a cognition enhancer. Serotonin is another regulator of emotion, among many other functions: one of the most consistent findings in the whole of biological psychiatry is that people with low levels of serotonin in their brains are less able to control impulses and are (therefore?) more likely to commit suicide.

Research on these chemical transmission systems tends to get bogged down in detail partly because they are so complicated (dopamine has at least four different types of receptor with differing functions, while the other two monoamines have more still), and partly because they are entangled; for example, the street drug LSD, which causes hallucinations, has its strongest direct effects on serotonin transmission, not on dopamine systems which appear to play the major part in most hallucination.

There is vastly more information about the neurotransmitters now than there was, say, twenty-five years ago and some previously unknown ones with very important roles have been discovered (e.g. NMDA). Nevertheless, it is probably harder now than it was then to discern any organising principles behind their variety or to explain why there should be such enormous complication.When physicists had only a few fundamental particles to worry about, they were probably happier than when particles started to proliferate in their cyclotrons. There is nothing in neurochemistry equivalent to the gauge theories that have helped physicists to sort out their burgeoning particles, though the relationship of neurotransmitters to brain function is in some ways analogous to that of fundamental particles to the structure of matter.

INFORMATION PROCESSING

This is what the brain does all the time and constitutes its *raison d'être*, so many people would say. It must do this processing in order to predict what is likely to happen next and cause the body to take appropriate action. A theologian might disagree, arguing that the brain's highest purpose is to know and to glorify God but, on pragmatic grounds, information processing has to be allowed precedence. All the more surprising, therefore, that consciousness is so little involved. Huge amounts of information reach the brain every instant, but of all this information only about seven items can be dealt with consciously. This begs a question about what an 'instant' might be (we shall postpone dealing with this question until the next Chapter). It is also not quite the same as saying that only seven bits of information can occupy awareness simultaneously since the 'items' may be complex; for instance one may be trying to decide which of seven symphonies one likes best, holding each of them in some sort of quasi-awareness for comparison. Psychologists point out that people can hold only around seven random digits in awareness simultaneously, and in these circumstances the content of awareness is limited to very few bits. To quote Nicolis and Tsuda (1985)

> the [conscious] channel which is so narrow and so noisy (of the order of just a few bits per second or a few bits per category) possesses the ability of squeezing . . . practically an unlimited number of bits per symbol – thereby giving rise to a phenomenal memory.

Despite the memory potential, most of what reaches the brain never gets into awareness.

Marcel, a psychologist working in Cambridge, has carried out a remarkable series of experiments on the relationship between conscious experience and automatic, non-conscious perception. Some of the more intriguing concern words with more than one meaning. You can show a word to someone without his being aware of it if it is very briefly flashed onto a screen and is quickly followed by another word. This is called 'masking'. If you show two words in succession that have related meanings (e.g. HAND followed by WRIST), people find it easier to classify the second. The trick is then to interpolate an ambiguous word. If PALM is used and is masked, it will assist classification of WRIST even if the first word shown is not HAND but TREE. If PALM is not masked so that the person is aware of it, it impairs classification of WRIST when the first word shown is TREE.

On the basis of work like this, Marcel (1983) concluded:

All sensory data impinging however briefly upon receptors sensitive to them is analysed, transformed, and redescribed, automatically and quite independently of consciousness, from its source form into every other representational form that the organism is capable of representing. This process of redescription will proceed to the highest and most abstract levels within the organism. Further, within every domain of redescription, wherever more than one parsing is possible of the data presented to it, all possible parsings will be carried out and represented . . . becoming conscious of something is merely like opening a door to, or it being pushed by, one aspiring entrant (out of many possible entrants).

The surprise is that so little of all that goes on gets into awareness, at least in a remememberable form. In this connection Polanyi (1964) had already pointed out that, when we are exploring the interior of a hole with a stick, we are aware of the shape of the hole but not the pressures of the stick on our hand even though it is only such pressures that give information about the hole.

The main point is that awareness alights on only a small proportion of brain activity, usually of the more abstract sort, though this is not always the case. When typing, for example, it is perfectly possible to be so aware of spelling and layout that one loses all track of meaning. Moreover, some of Marcel's work indicates that the apparent narrowness of awareness is real and is not simply due to inability to recall most conscious experience. One could not, for example, account for the opposite effects of an unconsciously and a consciously perceived PALM solely in terms of impaired recall.

It is generally thought nowadays that the brain uses parallel distributed processing in 'neural networks' to deal with information, not the sequential processing in a central processor typical of digital computers (see Bechtel and Abrahamsen, 1991). This neatly accounts for how many alternative interpretations of a single event can be simultaneously available to the brain, but of course creates a puzzle over why only one interpretation should usually enter awareness. If awareness was a simple epiphenomenon of information processing, the output of all parallel channels should surely enter it.

As mentioned previously, much of the information in the brain is entered as spatially organised sketches or maps of features of the world, though this may not always be the case. The posterior parietal cortex, for example, may through the spatial arrangement of its interconnections represent the rules by which different sensory maps can be converted into appropriate patterns to guide activity in motor maps controlling muscle activity (Stein, 1991). The fact that nervous activity in these various maps and other representations is probably chaotic (see, for example, Skarda and Freeman, 1987, or Lutzenberger *et al.*, 1992) does not really help one to understand the restricted range of awareness. Certainly, nervous activity over wide areas will come to be entrained by one or more of the 'strange attractors' of chaos theory, and different attractors may well represent different percepts or interpretations but, given that the Marcel experiments show that several of these can coexist, the question of why not all of them enter awareness again arises. If it could be answered we should probably have a good idea of what awareness is.

EXOTICA

It has seemed clear to neuroscientists for many years that information in the brain resides in patterns of activity in neurones, or in records of past patterns of such activity. Although neurone firing depends on neurotransmitter chemicals, their release is in turn due to depolarisation which is a form of electrical current flow. Ultimately, therefore, information depends on ion movements which entail electron movements. Once we are down to electrons, we have left behind the realm of classical physics and have entered that of quantum mechanics, of which more in Chapter 3. Penrose and others have pointed out that awareness can certainly be influenced by single quantum events since, in the right circumstances, the arrival of only one or two photons at the eye can cause a sensation of light. It is worth noting in this connection that, because of positional uncertainties, electrons can 'tunnel' across what ought to be an insulating junction thus making electric current flows in the brain less predictable than might be supposed. So far this will be familiar enough, at least to regular *New Scientist* readers. What may not be so familiar is that quantum particles other than electrons might occur in the brain which are in an even better position to act as information carriers.

Every form of energy has its particle aspect, according to quantum theory. Although the voltage across nerve cell membranes is small, they are so thin that the field gradients are very large (about 100,000 volts per centimetre). This is large enough to supply a lot of vibrational energy to any dipole molecules embedded in the cell membrane. There is good evidence that this form of energy is responsible for a phenomenon entirely familiar to all doctors; that is, the tendency of red blood cells to clump together (Rowlands, 1983). The particulate aspect of this energy is called a phonon, and this will be produced as depolarisation waves sweep along the cell membrane. Another type of vibrational energy that may be relevant is elastic deformation of chains of molecules, the particle aspect of which is called a Davydov soliton. Such chains (microtubules) form a major part of the structure of nerve cell processes, and it is interesting that the energy required to produce a soliton is about the same as that generated by hydrolysis of a molecule of ATP – the power source for all cellular processes. Therefore, solitons should frequently occur in neurones. Del Giudice *et al.* (1986) have given a most fascinating account of these various possibilities and have also pointed out that solitons ought to be capable of generating phonon type activity in water adhering to protein molecules. Water in this condition has most peculiar properties; for instance it freezes in the range -70° to -50° C and is a *bad* solvent for electrolytes.

Even more exotic are the massless particles which can be created by breaking symmetry of activity in neural nets. These are called Goldstone modes or bosons (Pessa, 1988). All these particles (phonons, solitons and Goldstone bosons) are potentially of great interest as they may be able to 'condense' (see Chapter 3) to produce large-scale objects in the brain which could take on a variety of topological shapes (see, for example, Wadati *et al.*, 1978 or Matsumoto *et al.*, 1979).

The likelihood that these entities exist may not seem very relevant until one recalls that spatial arrangement plays such a very important part in brain activity. After all, electrical activity is just the same in a neurone in the parietal cortex as in an occipital cortex neurone, so one can only account for the fact that the first gives rise to, say, awareness of a touch on one's hand and the other to a flash of light by referring to their different positions and interconnections. Goldstone bosons or the like may directly create a unified structure containing vital positional information. Brain activity is not necessarily only a matter of depolarisation waves and neurotransmitter release, it may have more important if less familiar components.

A most intriguing suggestion has been made by a leading researcher on anaesthetics who is based in Arizona (Hameroff, 1993). He pointed out that single cell organisms like *Paramecium* show complicated behaviours normally thought to require a brain of some sort, such as correctly aligning themselves with a potential mate, but they do it without benefit of a single synapse. It seems likely that their cellular skeleton, made up of microtubules, is their 'brain'. He goes on to argue that microtubules are quasi-crystals in which shape changes of the constituent protein (tubulin) could perform computational functions which would inherently involve quantum mechanical principles. The same considerations, of course, should apply to all cells, including those of our brains. It is a particularly nice idea as it roots the physical basis of cognition, and so possibly of awareness, in the basic structure of all animal cells, thus allowing one to see how it could have evolved into ever more elaborate forms.

THE UNCONSCIOUS

This heading is here mainly because people might expect it in a work of this sort. Actually, the notion of the unconscious is such a jumble, additionally confused by a lot of mistaken ideas derived from Freud, as to be unusable in the context of this book. The concept contains elements of innate and acquired predisposition, material that was never consciously registered, material that has been submerged by more recent events, stuff that is actively repressed and the constituents of fantasies that were never real. Much, perhaps most, brain activity is certainly not conscious, though we don't know what the proportion is because of the problem over recall of awareness mentioned in the introduction. However, introducing an entity called 'the unconscious' would only confuse matters.

To help track down awareness, we shall switch from thinking about its habitat to looking at its behaviour. The circumstances in which it changes form or begins to break down may provide insights into its nature. Some of these circumstances are part of normal experience, others due to illness.

SLEEP

People tend to think of themselves as habitually losing consciousness for eight hours, or whatever, out of every twenty-four. This is not in fact the case. What happens is that we lose immediate awareness of events in the external world, we lose the sensation of being able to direct our attention at will and we have few clear memories of what we experienced while we were asleep. However, people woken up from so-called rapid eye movement (REM) sleep always report awareness of vivid mental activity (dreams), and even those woken from slow wave sleep often recall awareness of having been engaged in cogitation or the like. Moreover, unusual percepts do tend to get through and are often woven into the material of dreams – most people, when a blanket has slipped off their feet in cold weather, will have had the experience of dreaming that they were wading through snow or something of that sort.

It's not worth speculating here about the functions of sleep which remain unknown, though clearly of great importance. To introduce a Darwinian argument of a type which will figure in future chapters, it may have been helpful to the survival of our ancestors to remain tucked up in trees during the hours of darkness, safe from predators, but sleep must be very risky for gnus, more at risk from hyenas at night than lions during the day, or dolphins for that matter who can get eaten by killer whales at any hour of day or night. Yet both these species still sleep; they mitigate the risks in the case of gnus by sleeping standing up in snatches of twenty minutes at a time while neighbours are awake, and in the case of dolphins, it is alleged, by allowing only one brain hemisphere at a time to doze off leaving the other alert. It therefore seems likely that sleep plays some essential part in brain housekeeping but is not of direct relevance to awareness.

What is relevant is the evidence from dreaming that brain activity of a different sort from the waking type is accompanied by awareness even though most of the awareness cannot be recalled for long. During REM sleep, brain energy use is as great or greater than during wakefulness, though it is somewhat reduced during slow wave sleep. Perhaps the vividness of REM dreams is a reflection of the energy involved. More surprising is the fact that there should be any awareness during slow wave sleep when the EEG (electro-encephalogram) activity is completely different from that seen during wakefulness. Awareness itself is evidently tolerant of very different electrical functional states of the brain, though its content and memorability are related to these functional states.

HYSTERICAL AND RELATED PHENOMENA

In the older psychiatric textbooks there were usually descriptions of people who, without any physical disease of the brain, would suddenly become blind, say, or lose the use of a limb. This was termed conversion hysteria. In these circumstances it was almost always possible to find some background story that made sense of the symptom. The blind person, for instance, might have witnessed some terrible accident in which a friend was killed, or someone with a paralysed arm might have experienced an overwhelming but wholly unacceptable urge to hit a parent. Crude symptoms like this rarely occur in educated populations these days, though more subtle ones of the same sort are not uncommon. They can still be found quite readily, however, in peasant societies.

One of the best ways of differentiating these disabilities from loss of function due to brain disease is to watch how the person behaves when his/her attention is not on the disability. Someone with hysterical blindness may truthfully say that he cannot see a hand held in front of his nose, but if a knife is flourished at him unexpectedly he will probably flinch; an hysterically paralysed arm cannot be moved by any effort of the patient's will, but if he trips over something accidentally it will move just as fast as the other arm to save him.

These symptoms can take incredibly elaborate forms. Multiple personality, for instance, is probably basically a hysterical phenomenon since it is very rare outside North America and is thus likely to be a creation of the American psychiatric culture. We all have somewhat different personae in different settings; the compliant yes-man at work who is a domestic tyrant has become a cliché. We all have fantasy personalities (e.g. the factory worker who is a brain surgeon in his daydreams) and these tend to be better developed in unhappy or traumatised people. In multiple personality, different personae take on separate lives and memories so that there is an appearance of different people sharing the same body. In the hands of therapists who do not think it a hysterical phenomenon, patients tend to acquire ever more personalities as time passes – the record number in a single patient is something like 40!

What appears to be happening in these cases is a breakdown in the expected range or unity of consciousness. Awareness is absent from the visual cortex of someone with hysterical blindness; it fails to link will and motor cortex in paralysis; memories and behaviours are fragmented in multiple personality. As we shall see later, this is often a consequence of brain disease or injury but the fact that it can occur in the absence of any organic dysfunction would seem to be a strong argument for the existence of some form of neurological/mental dualism. As usual, however, one cannot be precise about what may be going on because of uncertainty about whether awareness itself is restricted or fragmented, or whether it is simply a matter of selective suppression of recall of some aspects of awareness. Even in the case of the paralysis, one might argue that movement could not be voluntarily initiated because the relevant brain centres had been induced to forget how to go about it.

Some rather weak indications about underlying processes can be gained from considering what goes on during hypnosis. Incidentally, the fact that hypnosis can occur at all might be regarded as evidence that intentionality is not necessarily an integral part of an individual person's awareness but can reside elsewhere. A hypnotised person is aware, or at least he can report awareness just like the rest of us, but in a deep enough trance all intentionality in his awareness can appear to reside in the consciousness of the hypnotiser. On the other hand it might be argued that, in such circumstances, the two people are in some sense sharing a single consciousness so the intentionality is still integral. As we shall see later, there are views about the nature of awareness which give a basis for thinking that a consciousness which can be regarded as single may sometimes occupy more than one brain.

Getting back to the main theme of this section, which concerns fragmentation rather than transpersonal integration of consciousness, it is possible in good hypnotic subjects to induce states which appear identical to those seen in conversion hysteria; for all practical purposes they probably are identical. For instance, hysterical anaesthesia (inability to feel pain) can be mimicked. In one anecdote, a hypnotised person was told to bathe his tired feet in some lovely cool water. They were in fact put into uncomfortably hot water. 'Oh, how nice and refreshing this is', said the person. He had also been given some paper to write on: 'Ouch! this hurts' said his hand. It is difficult to account for this sort of story in terms of selective recall impairment; awareness may truly be fragmented. However, all experiments with hypnosis have to be taken with a pinch of salt since it is so easy for the experimenter to quite unwittingly influence his subject to produce the answer that he wants.

PSYCHOSIS

What happens in psychotic illnesses shows that awareness can be filled, even when a person is awake, with material that has nothing to do with the real world (hallucinations), or can become fragmented or distorted in various unusual ways. Hallucinations in one of the commonest of these illnesses, schizophrenia, are usually rather dull. Unreal voices, that seem entirely real to the sufferer, mumbling obscenities or repeating the person's thoughts out loud are common and cause much distress. But they can be vivid and enthralling; one patient who used to talk to me regularly has for fifteen years had such enthralling 'telepathic' experiences involving all sorts of aliens, gods and people that he refuses to take the medication which would remove his symptoms (he tried it once and found it effective) because everyday life is so dull by comparison.

Hallucinations are often particularly vivid in deliria due to some general disease of the body. It says in most textbooks that these deliria are accompanied by 'clouding' of consciousness, but this is not at all obvious in some cases who can appear just as alert as anyone else. Here are a couple of examples:

A self-employed builder had been raised on a farm but was living in a suburban street at the time he became ill. He was in the habit of drinking about 12 pints of Guinness a day. One day he decided that this might be a bit too much and that he should give it up. Unfortunately for him, delirium tremens can be brought on by *withdrawal* of excess alcohol. The following morning, he woke up, dressed and had breakfast as usual, then stepped out of his front door into a field of ripe, waving barley that obviously needed harvesting. He tried to get passers by to help with the harvest and could not understand why they were unwilling. Then he stopped the cars which were trying to drive over the field – and of course got taken into custody. One can, perhaps, argue that in his case some stored childhood memory had become inappropriately activated and had somehow 'taken over'.

It's less easy to account for the experience of my grandfather during a long illness when he was aged 86, though not at all senile. He spent long, happy hours writing articles for Canadian newspapers and saw these projected on to the wall in front of his bed. He was very appreciative of the new technology which achieved this projection and saved him the bother of typing. However, he had been an MP, not a journalist, and had visited Canada only once, briefly and about forty years previously.

A vivid example of the way in which awareness can become fragmented is provided by the so-called Capgras syndrome which can form part of a schizophrenic illness. The patient becomes convinced that relatives and friends have been replaced by impostors. 'Yes, I know she looks exactly like my mother', the patient will say, 'but it's not really her, it's some stranger that has taken her over'. This is presumably a reflection of the fact that brain centres for recognising faces are separate from those storing emotional responses to our nearest and dearest. The two normally give rise to an integrated experience, but the integration can break down. Incidentally, the opposite phenomenon can occur; people can become convinced that complete strangers have been taken over by the essence of those close to them. Inappropriate integration of awareness, it seems, can also occur.

Similar inappropriate integration, in a more general form, is often found in severe depression. In this condition a pervasive mood of misery, despair and hopelessness can get attached to all sorts of extraneous circumstances, so that a person may wrongly come to believe that they have a fatal disease, or are about to become bankrupt, or their spouse is unfaithful. What is particularly interesting, from our point of view, is that the changes in the content of awareness in the psychoses are accompanied by changes in the use of energy by various parts of the brain.

REGIONAL ENERGY USE

The brain gets its energy from burning glucose with oxygen. Using a technique called PET scanning (Positron Emission Tomography), it is possible to get two-dimensional cross-sectional pictures of the brain 'shaded' according to how much glucose or oxygen is being consumed. The technique is similar to the better-known CAT scan (Computerised Axial Tomography) which uses X-rays and produces brain cross-sections shaded according to how dense, in the sense of how impenetrable to the X-rays, different areas are.

There are various problems with PET scanning, especially the cost and complexity of the apparatus needed. However, oxygen use is closely related to blood flow and there are several techniques for producing brain pictures which show this. They are xenon flow (the oldest, now largely superceded), SPET scanning (Single Photon Emission Tomography) and fast MRI (Magnetic Resonance Imaging). SPET is cheap and widely available. Fast MRI is very expensive but gives the most information as the picture resolution (the amount of detail shown) is far better and it can follow rapid changes in flow (of the order of a second or so). However, all the techniques produce roughly equivalent results and have been used to confirm each other's validity. They show that, when a particular brain area is being used, it uses more energy than the rest of the brain. Not very surprising, one might think, albeit a useful confirmation of previous conclusions about which brain areas serve what function. There have been some surprises, though. For instance, increased flow when using a hand can occur in a small area of the motor cortex on the *same* side as the hand, as well as on the expected opposite side. Increase in blood flow due to use of an area is of the order of 5 per cent to 30 per cent. (see David *et al.*, 1994, for a concise account of these findings).

A great many studies using these techniques have been carried out on psychotic patients, most of which show that they differ from normal people in the use of one or more brain areas, even though one study may show patients using a particular area more, another shows them using it less and yet another no difference. In general, people with schizophrenia show reduced use of their frontal lobes (usually with associated changes in parts of their corpora striata and thalami); if they have hallucinations or delusions, they will almost certainly have energy use changes in or around their left temporal lobes.

An especially interesting study of depressed people (Blench *et al.*, 1993) found that those who were anxious had increased blood flow on both sides in certain localised areas (posterior cingulate cortex and inferior parietal lobe), those who were slowed up and felt particularly low in mood had reduced flow in different areas (left dorsolateral prefrontal cortex and left angular gyrus), while people whose concentration was very impaired showed reduced flow in yet another area (medial prefrontal pole). The precise areas don't matter to non-specialists, so readers should not trouble to look them up. What is relevant is that the areas affected varied according to the symptoms experienced.

These and similar results extend earlier findings in psychotic patients using entirely different techniques (e.g. neuropsychological testing, brain electrical activity mapping). There can no longer be any doubt that particular brain areas specialise in particular emotional or cognitive functions just as different areas specialise in sight or movement. This is not to conclude that they work in isolation, as clearly they don't, but nevertheless separate emotional or cognitive happenings tend to arise from activity in separate brain areas. Also, having an emotion entails extra energy use by some particular brain area just as, say, opening one's eyes involves extra energy use by the visual cortex.

NEUROLOGICAL ABNORMALITIES

Head injuries and strokes have always provided valuable hints about which bits of the brain do what. If a stroke destroys the parietal lobe, say, sensation on the opposite side of the body will be lost, at least to start off with. If damage is confined to the primary sensory areas, the person will be aware that he's lacking awareness, but if association areas are also involved the patient may not notice anything amiss. Deficits can take bizarre forms, exemplified by the title of Oliver Sach's well-known collection of essays, *The Man Who Mistook His Wife for a Hat.* A problem with trying to extend this sort of approach into getting evidence about subtle aspects of function is that one is never quite sure whether changes in awareness, or other symptoms, are due to loss of the brain area that has been destroyed or to overactivity of other areas which were previously inhibited by the damaged part.

The opposite approach, stimulating selected brain areas into overactivity with an electrical probe, is a bit more reliable. It was used for many years, from the 1930s to the 1960s, by Wilder Penfield, a Canadian neurosurgeon. He made systematic observations on conscious patients whose brains were exposed in the course of operations for tumours and severe epilepsy. His work is the main foundation for much of our knowledge about localisation of brain function. It was regarded as ethical at the time it was done because it was in any case an essential part of each patient's treatment that they should be probed while able to report on their experiences (in order to determine how extensive an operation was required for their particular condition). Nowadays greater sensitivity about what constitutes valid consent, the need to minimise operating time and other issues means that similar work is usually thought unethical in all but the most exceptional circumstances. Perhaps the most interesting finding, from the point of view of thinking about awareness, was the variability of experience dependent on the brain area stimulated. Stimulating some areas produced a quale, usually a fairly crude one; a flash of light if it was the visual cortex, say, or a sensation of reaching for something if it was a motor association area. A more complex experience, hearing a snatch of song, for instance, could sometimes be got from the temporal lobes. But from many areas stimulation elicited no awareness whatsoever. It seems that an awareness can result from artificial brain stimulation, as indeed we all know from 'seeing stars' after hitting our heads, but it does not necessarily do so.

There was a great deal of excitement in the 1970s over 'split-brain' patients. These were people who had had the main fibre tract (the corpus callosum) between the two hemispheres of the brain divided as a treatment for otherwise incurable epilepsy. All sorts of ingenious methods were devised for communicating with and testing each half of the brain independently. Not altogether surprisingly, the two halves tended to behave independently, at least for a time after the operation, since their habitual communication link with each other had been destroyed. For instance, if a picture of a nude was shown to the right hemisphere only, causing the patient to give a sly grin, his left hemisphere and so his speech centres might have no knowledge of the cause of the grin, and would make up some rationalisation when asked to account for it. People speculated about whether the operation had created two minds or persons sharing a single body; some suggested that only the left hemisphere has true consciousness and the right hemisphere is nothing but a neurological computer – this in marked contrast to other 1970s writers who were claiming that the logical left hemisphere is the robot and we should all cultivate our holistic and intuitive right hemispheres!

Elementary facts tended to get submerged in all the brouhaha; for instance that the patients only had the operation because of severe pre-existing brain dysfunction and this may have been responsible for some of their difficulties on testing. Occasionally, people are born without a corpus callosum and they don't seem to provide nearly such striking findings as the patients; one can argue that they have had time to develop alternative communication channels which is probably correct since the patients themselves tend to improve with time. These findings have provided some interesting technical information about the functions of the corpus callosum, but it is hard to see that they tell us anything fundamental about the nature of mentality or personality that we did not already know from observation of stroke victims and the like.

A more recent focus of interest has been the phenomenon called 'blindsight'. People whose primary visual cortex has been destroyed (by stroke, injury or tumour – there are no wicked surgeons wantonly damaging healthy people) say they cannot see anything at all. When tested, however, they can detect visual stimuli in the sense that they can point to where a light is, or distinguish between round and triangular objects. What the experimenter usually does is ask the patient to guess and he then gets it right while claiming he can see nothing. The standard explanation is that the patient succeeds by making use of those visual pathways that don't go to the visual cortex and that such tracts do not involve consciousness. Unfortunately, of course, it could equally well be the case that the alternative visual tracts do not have the right memory mechanisms to allow report of any awareness in them. It's intriguing that, with time and practise, people do tend to get crude visual sensations, for instance 'a feeling of roughness' in response to an irregular object shown to them. This could be due to consciousness starting to occur in previously unconscious pathways, or to recovery starting to happen in the visual cortex, or to the beginnings of memory for previously unremembered awareness in alternative pathways. As no one has devised a way of distinguishing between these alternatives, blindsight, too, has less to tell us about consciousness than has sometimes been claimed.

Finally, it's worth pointing out that there is confirmation of the assumption that it is the brain *cortex*, i.e. the surface of the brain, and brain stem that subserve awareness and cognition, while the bulk of the white matter in the cerebral hemispheres may not be all that important. There are fluid filled cavities in the brain and these can sometimes become much larger than normal, producing a condition called hydrocephalus. If this enlargement happens very gradually as a child is growing up, it may go completely unnoticed. Several cases have been reported where most of the insides of the cerebral hemispheres were found to have been replaced by fluid, leaving only a thin rind of cortex plastered against the skull. This is apparently compatible with having normal intelligence and living a normal life; indeed one such case was a successful architect. The evidence that the brain stem is important comes from findings (e.g. Heimer, 1983) that crude awarenesses, especially of pain, can occur in the absence of relevant cortical areas provided the thalamus is intact.

CONCLUSIONS

This rapid survey of aspects of the brain has shown that it is a sort of patchwork quilt of structures, functions and chemical transmitters. We don't generally notice the seams, but they become only too obvious in the course of both mental and neurological illnesses, and also when one applies certain research techniques. Awareness seems to light almost capriciously on a tiny proportion of total brain activity. One can perfectly well be occupied with admiring a flower, while unaware that parts of one's mind are solving a crossword clue or planning tomorrow's dinner menu. Of course attention, which we have hitherto ignored, plays a large part in directing the flow of conscious experience but this, too, can be subject to awareness or can operate unconsciously. Attention is just another brain function that can be shown to have localised manifestations (mainly in the frontal lobes) which may or may not enter awareness.

It is almost as if the creature we are seeking (awareness) was a sort of butterfly flitting from patch to patch of the brain quilt, just like the heraldic image of the psyche. Are we in a position yet to say anything useful about it? An important observation is that awareness can survive in the absence of the normal external inputs to the brain, since dreams occur and hallucinations can be as vivid as everyday reality. As the Penfield experiments show, it can be artificially induced to alight on particular bits of patchwork. We also got a hint that it might be tolerant of quite widely differing electrical functional states of the brain. However, it was a rather uncertain hint as it depended on reports of consciousness during slow wave sleep, and of course the reports could only be made after waking. Perhaps awareness can falsely attribute consciousness to memories of what was in fact unconscious activity. There is no end to the difficulties caused by uncertainty over the possible role(s) of memory, but at least the Marcel experiments give some assurance that genuinely unconscious brain activity does occur – it's not all a matter of having forgotten awareness.

Two main themes seem to have emerged in relation to our butterfly; first, its energy requirements, second, the essential links that shape and position have with it. Its energy needs are high, as one could have inferred simply from the fact that choking someone renders them unconscious quite a while before irreparable nerve cell damage is done. But what is it that needs so much energy? Depolarisation waves and neurotransmitter release are going on all the time in all brain areas, but where awareness occurs blood flow requirements suddenly increase by up to 30 per cent. No doubt this is because there are increased rates of nerve cells firing in brain areas that are undertaking some specific task. All the same, it's not obvious why depolarisation waves occurring at the rate of 10/sec., say, should not be associated with awareness in contrast to those occurring at 50/sec. Maybe faster firing rates are associated with more widespread activity, or more complex feedback, or something of that sort.

We have, however, found another candidate for the substrate of awareness which has clearly defined high energy needs. That is the potential condensate among phonons or other quasi-particles. The whole subject will be dealt with at length later on, but it's worth saying at this stage that phonons have attracted more interest than the other two types of particle (solitons and Goldstone bosons). There's a problem with them as Clarke (1994) has found theoretical evidence that the energy spectrum is too widespread to allow condensation among phonons in nerve cell membranes. Tubulin-associated phonons, fortunately, may be in a better position to condense as the associated energy will tend to get channelled by the microtubules and so will be confined to a narrower range (Hameroff, 1993). An explanation of the term 'condensation' will be given in Chapter 3.

The importance of shape to awareness is evident at all levels from the effect of anaesthetics on the shape of protein molecules to the 'maps' which are so vital to cortical function. To repeat an earlier comment, there is no inherent difference in electrical activity between an occipital neurone and a parietal one, so it is only possible to account for the different experiences to which stimulating them will give rise in terms of their position within different overall patterns of activity. It is also clear that some patterns provide a sort of reflection of features of the external world. However, we have gained no clear ideas, yet, about what awareness has to do with these ghostly shapes within the brain, or indeed about what defines a unified pattern. Hypothetical condensates may provide the beginnings of some sort of answer; but again, they may not. It's time to move on to thinking about the temporal aspects of brain function.

REFERENCES

Bechtel, W. and Abrahamsen, A. (1991) *Connectionism and the Mind*, Basil Blackwell: Oxford.

Berridge, C.W., Arnsten, A.F.T. and Foote, S.L. (1993) 'Editorial: Noradrenergic Modulation of Cognitive Function', *Psychological Medicine* 23, 557–64.

Blench, C.J., Friston, K.J., Brown, R.G., Frackowiak, R.S.J. and Dolan, R.J. (1993) 'Regional Cerebral Blood Flow in Depression Measured by PET: The Relationship with Clinical Dimensions', *Psychological Medicine* 23, 579–90.

Clarke, C.J.S. (1994) 'Coupled Molecular Oscillators Do Not Admit True Bose Condensations' (to appear in *Journal of Physics A.*).

David, A., Blamire, A. and Breiter, H. (1994) 'Editorial: Functional Magnetic Resonance Imaging', *British Journal of Psychiatry* 164, 2–7.

Del Giudice, E., Doglia, S., Milani, M. and Vitiello, G. (1986) 'Collective Properties of Biological Systems: Solitons and Coherent Electric Waves in a Quantum Field Theoretical Approach', in *Modern Bioelectrochemistry*, F. Gutmann and H. Keyzer (eds), Plenum: New York.

DeMott, D.W. (1970) *Toposcopic Studies of Learning*, Charles C. Thomas: Springfield, Illinois.

Edelman, G.M. (1989) *The Remembered Present: A Biological Theory of Consciousness*, Basic Books: New York.

Franks, N.P. and Lieb, W.R. (1994) 'Molecular and Cellular Mechanisms of General Anaesthesia', *Nature* 367, 607–13.

Hameroff, S.R. (1993) 'Quantum Conformational Automata in the Cytoskeleton: Nanoscale Cognition in Protein Connectionist Networks', Preprint for conference report, *Towards a Material Basis for Cognition*, Abisko (Sweden).

Heimer, L. (1983) *The Human Brain and Spinal Chord*, Springer-Verlag: New York.

Lutzenberger, W., Elbert, T., Birbaumer, N., Ray, W.J. and Schupp, H. (1992) 'The Scalp Distribution of the Fractal Dimension of the EEG and its Variation with Mental Tasks', *Brain Topography* 5 (1), 27–33.

Marcel, A.J. (1983) 'Conscious and Unconscious Perception: An Approach to the Relations between Phenomenal Experience and Perceptual Processes', *Cognitive Psychology* 15, 238–300.

Matsumoto, H., Sodano, P. and Umezawa, H. (1979) 'Extended Objects in Quantum Systems and Soliton Solutions', *Physical Review D.* 19, 511–15.

Nedergaard, M. (1994) 'Direct Signalling from Astrocytes to Neurones in Cultures of Mammalian Brain Cells', *Science* 263, 1768–71.

Nicolis, J.S. and Tsuda, I. (1985) 'Chaotic Dynamics of Information Processing: The "Magic Number Seven Plus-Minus Two" Revisited', *Bulletin of Mathematical Biology* 47 (3), 343–65.

Pessa, E. (1988) 'Symmetry Breaking in Neural Nets', *Biological Cybernetics* 59, 277–81.

Polanyi, M. (1964) *Personal Knowledge: Towards a Post-Critical Philosophy*, Harper: New York.

Rowlands, S. (1983) 'Coherent Excitations in Blood', in *Coherent Excitations in Biological Systems*, H. Frohlich and F. Kremer (eds), Springer-Verlag: Berlin.

Skarda, C.A. and Freeman W.J. (1987) 'How Brains Make Chaos in Order to Make Sense of the World', *Behavioural and Brain Sciences* 10, 161–95.

Stein, J.F. (1991) 'Space and Parietal Association Areas', in *Brain and Space*, J. Paillard (ed.), Oxford University Press.

Wadati, M., Matsumoto, H. and Umezawa H. (1978) 'Extended Objects Created by Goldstone Bosons', *Physical Review D.* 18, 520–31.

2 Time and awareness

Awareness exists in time as well as in some sort of 'space' within the brain, so there's not much hope of understanding consciousness without a knowledge of how time, brain and awareness are related. Unfortunately, it's a slippery subject to tackle for a wide range of reasons. One fairly basic difficulty is that we have no adequate vocabulary with which to discuss it. Take that catch phrase used by trendy managers in the early 1980s – 'At this moment in time'. It seems fairly innocuous at first hearing, if ugly and trite, until one dwells on what 'moment' might mean. To a relativity theorist it would probably imply a minimum quantum unit of duration taking in all events occurring on the surface of a light cone originating from the manager who spoke; not a very helpful concept for everyday purposes.

A subjective moment is a variable entity. When faced with some disaster that one cannot avoid, in a skidding car with a wall looming for instance, quite small fractions of a second can be indelibly etched on one's awareness. If relaxed in a comfortable chair with music playing in the background, ten seconds or more can form a single instant. It's probably helpful to think of two different types of moment; first, the minimum perceptual duration of around 0.1 second which is always in the background, but can be experienced consciously in circumstances of extreme arousal; next, the so-called specious present which corresponds to our usual experience of a moment and normally has a duration of anywhere between about 1 and 15 seconds.

Lockwood (1989: Chapter 15) points out that there is a problem with the idea of the specious present best illustrated by thinking about one's experience of music. Several notes, even a whole tune, can be experienced as a single quale occupying an extended moment, but the experience depends on an awareness of the succession of notes, thus implying the occurrence of a succession of experiential sub-moments. It seems at first sight to be a paradox, and Lockwood's preferred resolution of it is somewhat involved. However, he neglects the evidence that there are nerve cells, in the temporal lobes of the brain appropriately enough, which become active in relation to the order in which particular stimuli arrive at the brain. When awareness includes the activity in these cells their information gets incorporated in the resultant quale, just as information about the colour of the pianist's face or one's emotional reaction to the music may also be incorporated. There is in fact no paradox. This interpretation implies that perception always has some duration, but this is hardly contentious as there is no perception without at least one neural depolarisation wave and such waves have a duration.

The sensation of the passage of time has been described quite elegantly by Brown (1990: 144) in the passage quoted below. It's not an account that provides any easily accessible intellectual illumination, but does give a good description of the background to the 'feel' of what goes on:

> Mind transforms the continuance of physical spacetime into moments. . . and blends these moments into an apparent continuity through an overlapping of unfolding capsules. Each mind computes the measure of time passing and duration from the decay of the surface present in relation to a core of past events. As each new surface is generated, that surface, the rim of the immediate past, recedes in the wake of rising contents. This recession, an uncovering of phases latent in the original traversal, exposes layers in the past forming the content of the immediate past moment. The surge of the microgeny to a surface that dissolves the instant it appears, the priority of the Self in the unfolding sequence, the feeling of agency, create a Self in a process of becoming, a Self that travels *in time* like the crest of a wave, always in pursuit of a future just beyond the grasp of the present.

MINIMUM PERCEPTUAL DURATION

Any computer has to have a clock so that computations can be related to one another, and dealt with in an orderly sequence in the case of machines with a central processor. The rate at which the clock ticks is usually described in units referred to as Hz (1 Hz or hertz = 1 cycle per second). The faster the clock ticks in a sequential computer, the faster it can operate and even quite cheap machines are now regarded as slow if their clocks work at 'only' 16 MHz (1 megahertz = 1 million cycles per second). The brain, too, contains a range of clocks some of which tick slowly, tied to the twenty-four hour day/night cycle or even the changing seasons. Others are faster, though it's not known how fast they get. It used to be supposed that information in the brain was coded in average rates of depolarisation waves occurring over a period of time. This implied that the fastest clocks had nevertheless to be slow enough for averages to have time to accrue between ticks. However, Gerstner *et al.* (1993) have recently provided cogent theoretical reasons for supposing that neural networks deal with information far more efficiently if it is coded in patterns of single depolarisation waves rather than the average rates of sequences of waves. If correct this would require a brain clock working at up to 1000 Hz.

There is quite good evidence for the existence of a brain clock working at around 10 Hz (e.g. Nunn and Osselton, 1974). This particular machine may in some ways be analogous to the shutter of a cine-camera which is also, of course, a sort of clock. Each tick appears to prevent information reaching, or being processed by, sensory areas just as shutter closure in a camera stops light reaching the film. The idea is that, in some important respects, the brain deals with time-bounded packages of information each lasting around 0.1 seconds. This may be the minimum 'chunk' of information that can be consciously perceived and would normally contain the famous seven items which are the maximum that can be held in awareness at any given moment (see Chapter 1).

This is a particularly attractive possibility from the point of view of a psychiatrist as it allows one to construct a simple model that accounts for much of the phenomenology of all the so-called 'functional' psychoses (Nunn, 1980). There are plenty of theories about why schizophrenic symptoms take the form that they do, and others that account for mania or depression, but this is unique in having something to say about all three. It can also accommodate intermediate forms of psychosis and account for the hallucinations that occasionally result from sleep deprivation and sensory deprivation. It depends basically on Murphy's law (anything that can go wrong will sometimes go wrong). A shutter in the brain will therefore sometimes fail to close properly or will sometimes let in too much or too little 'light'. Each of these possibilities, according to the model, corresponds to a different psychosis.

Actually, of course, it is too simple to do more than provide a hint about what may be going on in the brain. As mentioned in the previous Chapter, electrodes placed on the scalp or the surface of the cortex pick up rhythmic electrical changes due to net current flows in the underlying fluid and, to a lesser extent, prolonged voltage alterations in interwoven nerve cell processes. It's the old technique called electro-encephalography (EEG) first described by Berger between the World Wars. The best known of these rhythms, the alpha rhythm, has the right characteristics to be an expression of the activity of our 'brain shutter' since its frequency is around 10 Hz (it is defined as 8–13 Hz) and, overall, its amplitude decreases both if concentrating on something and if one drifts off to sleep. One can picture the shutter as being open for longer when concentrating and closed for longer when sleeping, so maximum contrast between open and shut phases will occur at awake but idle phases. The trouble is that there's not just one alpha rhythm but a great many with slightly differing frequencies, some of which vary with attention and others not. If a brain clock does exist that has some of the characteristics of a shutter, it is not the simple device that one might wish to picture – but then the brain is like that; it appears to take a perverse pleasure in apparently unnecessary complexity of design and function.

EEG TEMPORAL CODINGS

Rhythms that can be picked up in the EEG range from less than 1 Hz to more than 300 Hz. Their existence implies the occurrence of synchronised or correlated nerve cell activity beneath the recording electrodes, and a lot of interest has centred recently around determining whether EEG activity in separate areas of the brain is also correlated. This can be done by ascertaining whether frequency and phase changes of the EEG in, for instance, parts of the occipital cortex are sometimes related to those in parts of the frontal lobes or elsewhere. According to Cook (1991):

> the list of situations in which correlated activity is known or strongly suspected to be highly influential now embraces almost every branch of neuroscience, including perception, memory and the development and plasticity of structural and functional linkages throughout the Central Nervous System.

Although this sounds rather grand, it is really only a different way of saying that the activity of one nerve cell or group of cells often temporarily or permanently influences that of other parts of the brain, which we already knew. Its usefulness lies in the emphasis placed on EEG correlational studies as a research tool, plus the observation that correlation of activity between remote parts of the brain can develop fast, within a few tens of milliseconds.

There was much excitement a few years ago when it was discovered that areas of the brain that might be supposed to be engaged in a perceptual task of some sort showed episodes of correlated 40 Hz activity lasting for up to around half a second (Barinaga, 1990). Intervening brain areas not necessary for the task did not show the same activity. This finding has held up fairly well. Correlated activity consequent on task performance appears in widely separated patches of the brain, though it seems to occur not only at 40 Hz but over a wide frequency band (Bressler *et al.*, 1993).

There's a temptation to think that this solves the 'binding' problem of how activity in patches of cortex remote from each other combines to form a single quale. Maybe neurones that vibrate together are together in some important sense, and no doubt this is true. The trouble is that it's not obvious in what sense it might be true. The neurone groups remain spatially separated, and all that has been achieved is to show that temporally determined groupings are important to brain activity as well as spatially related groupings. In future it will be necessary to think of spatio-temporal functional units. This is an important step forward but it does not obviously get us any nearer towards accounting for awareness.

Evidence from a *magneto*encephalographic study (Salmelin *et al.*, 1994) suggests that the whole situation is more complicated than EEG coherence enthusiasts might like. It will be recalled that the MEG is sensitive to current flows along axon bundles, while the EEG is the outcome of a whole rag-bag of electrical phenomena. What Salmelin and co-workers did was to look at MEG activation while people were putting names to drawings of various objects. Activation was seen in the occipital cortex within 200 msecs of the drawing being shown, and it then spread forwards reaching fronto-temporal areas some 400 msecs later. Actual naming of the drawing began at 750 to 975 msecs There was no simultaneous activation appearing in remote areas subserving the whole naming process. 'So what?' one might say, 'This simply means that the EEG reflects processes underlying awareness and the MEG does not'. The problem is, though, that it is axonal current flows that are usually thought to reflect most closely information flow relevant to the content of consciousness. This is because axonal flows are directly driven by the depolarisation waves that are thought to encode information. It is far from clear what the correlated EEG activity is actually reflecting.

There's quite a bit of evidence that different EEG frequencies are especially associated with different sorts of brain activity, though there is probably quite a lot of overlap. Activity of 40 Hz certainly does seem to be especially related to perception along with higher frequencies of perhaps up to 120 Hz. This is not to say that these frequencies are necessarily involved in *conscious* perception; it's more likely that they reflect Marcel-type unconscious or pre-conscious functions.

It has long been thought (e.g. Ray and Cole, 1985) that alpha activity (defined variously as 8 to 12 or 13 Hz) reflects attention and beta activity (from 14 to 20 or 30 Hz; some authors refer to frequencies greater than 25 Hz as gamma activity) reflects cognitive and emotional functions. Even lower frequencies may also have their special associations. For instance, Basar-Eroglu *et al.* (1992) think that delta frequencies (3 Hz or less) are 'Mainly involved in signal matching, decision-making and surprise, whereas theta responses (4 to 7 Hz) are more related to focused attention and signal detection'. It's not surprising that there should be a good deal of overlap in assigned functions because activity in one frequency band is often related, directly or reciprocally, to that in another. All the same it is interesting that vital functions like attention and decision-making should be related to such low frequency 'clocks'. There would almost certainly be big evolutionary advantages in performing functions of this sort faster, if it were possible. A gazelle that could make decisions at 100 Hz would be a gazelle unlikely to be caught by any cheetah operating at 10 Hz, and the same would have applied to our ancestors. The fact that the clocks have remained low frequency probably means that they can't run faster. There must be some ill-understood design constraint analogous to that which has kept the main part of our brains two-dimensional. This could be a need to allow time for average rates of nerve cell firing to accrue but, if Gerstner and colleagues are right about the greater efficiency of patterns of single spikes, one would have expected evolution to have made use of them if there were no additional constraints.

EVOKED POTENTIALS

These are EEG events due to some specific stimulus. Because there is a lot of apparently random activity going on all the time in the EEG, you can't see the response to a flash of light, say, or a touch on one's leg; it gets swamped by everything else that is going on. But if repeated, identical stimuli are given and the EEG is taken and averaged after each, then the random fluctuations cancel out and the response to whatever stimulus it was can be seen plainly.

There are two main varieties of evoked potential, depending on different experimental set-ups. The less-used one was discovered by Grey Walter who worked in Bristol after the Second World War, and was responsible for the mechanical tortoise shown at the Festival of Britain which could trundle around avoiding obstacles and seek out an electric point to recharge itself when necessary; a great wonder at a time before transistors or printed circuits had been invented. He called his discovery an 'expectancy wave' which was accurate and vivid – it now goes by the dour and uninformative title of 'contingent negative variation', no doubt as a result of the current vogue for giving important things a three-word acronym where possible (cf. the transformation of head cooks into catering services managers).

What Grey Walter found was that if you asked someone to press a button after hearing a buzzer and then signalled that the buzzer was about to sound by turning on a light, a negative voltage change would appear, mainly over frontal areas, when the light went on that vanished when the person had pressed their button. Of course, the whole sequence had to be repeated many times, and the EEG signal averaged, in order to pick out the expectancy wave from all the clutter. This finding has remained a bit of a curiosity; there were attempts to use it to make psychiatric diagnoses since some patients have lower voltage waves than normal people, but these fizzled out as there was so much overlap between the patients and normals.

Sensory evoked potentials, however, have gone from strength to strength. They are much used as a diagnostic tool in neurology and a research tool in neuropsychiatry. All that they involve is giving a repeated, simple sensory stimulus and then averaging the EEGs recorded after each stimulus. Widely-used stimuli, affecting different sensory modalities, include clicks, small (non-painful) electric shocks to limbs and reversing the black and white squares on a chequerboard. The resultant EEG responses are a bit reminiscent of what happens when a stone is dropped into water. There is a localised 'plop' in the appropriate bit of sensory cortex, followed by spreading ripples of activity. It is thought that the later ripples (at around 300 or 400 msecs after the stimulus provoking them) reflect elaborations in dealing with the information in the stimulus and thus may be connected with consciousness. Basar (1992) has pointed out that the ripples don't just happen at any old frequency, but are related to the underlying 'natural' frequencies of the brain clocks.

THE LIBET EXPERIMENTS

According to A.N. Whitehead, who worked with Bertrand Russell at the turn of the century on 'Principia Mathematica' (that great work intended to derive all mathematics from a few axioms: a task later proved by Godel to be inherently impossible): 'Consciousness is the subjective form of an intellectual feeling which arises, if at all, only in the late phase of a moment of experience'. This may seem a silly statement; after all, consciousness surely exists only in the present moment. If it does not occur in the objective now, when on earth could it exist? As it turns out, however, Whitehead was being prescient, not silly at all. If one can criticise anything about his claim, it is his use of the word 'experience', which implies awareness, to refer to what is mostly unconscious or pre-conscious. 'Neural activity' would have made a better choice.

Over a period of more than thirty years, Benjamin Libet (1989, 1993), who works at the San Francisco School of Medicine, has carried out a series of elegant experiments on just when, and under what circumstances, consciousness occurs in relation to neural events. His research techniques have involved recording evoked potentials and using direct electrical stimulation of the brain similar to that employed by Wilder Penfield (Chapter 1). His findings are remarkable and worth describing in some detail.

As Penfield discovered, you can elicit a sensory experience by stimulating the appropriate neural pathway or area of primary sensory cortex. Libet found that in order to elicit an awareness from cortex or the tracts leading to it *above the spinal chord* the stimulus must both be greater than a certain intensity and last for a sufficient time of anything up to 500 msecs (1 msec. or millesecond is one-thousandth of a second). No stimulus, however intense, that was too brief would elicit a conscious experience. When stimulating nerves in the periphery or in the spinal chord, however, the stimulus had only to be above a certain intensity to elicit awareness. The necessary intensity is probably that sufficient to produce the longer-lasting 'ripples' of the evoked response. Large, short-lived local responses, adjacent to a stimulus site in the sensory cortex do not seem to matter; they can be produced by stimuli of insufficient intensity to give rise to awareness and can be abolished altogether (by applying an inhibitory neurotransmitter) without affecting awareness of more intense stimuli.

A further indication that it's long-lasting activity that matters was provided by finding that the sensation produced by a low intensity pulse to the skin could be enhanced by later stimulating the appropriate (somatosensory) bit of cortex. This enhancement occurred even when the cortical stimulation was delayed for 400 msecs after the skin pulse. All this appears to relate to *awareness*, not just information processing, as stimuli of insufficient intensity or duration to give rise to an awareness can still be shown to have been detected by giving an appropriate test, similar to the tests used on 'blindsight' patients. Moreover, one can make coherent reactions to things in around 100 or 200 msecs which is a lot less than the up to 500 msecs needed for awareness of them to develop.

How is it, then, that we seem to ourselves to be living in the present rather than in memories half a second old? Libet investigated this by the very ingenious method of giving people pulses to the skin and pulses to the sensory cortex at various time intervals, and then asking the people to judge which sensation came first or whether they were simultaneous. Sensations due to cortical stimulation were judged to occur after the stimulus had been going on for long enough to produce awareness, but those due to skin stimulation were judged to have happened when the first 'plop' due to the stimulus occurred in the cortex. In other words, sensations due to stimuli arriving naturally at the brain are *referred back in time* to the first arrival of information concerning them, even though the sensation itself takes up to half a second to develop. This process of backward referral appears to be entirely automatic and is incorporated as an integral part of the resultant quale. Although we are all living half a second behind the times, we seem to ourselves to dwell in the objective present. This seems startling, but it has of course been known for a long while that we live a bit behind the times because it takes a few milliseconds for information from one's skin, say, to reach one's central nervous system; it's just the size of the delay that is surprising.

Perhaps even more disconcerting are Libet's discoveries about voluntary acts. Potentials similar to Grey Walter's 'expectancy wave' occur before any act; even spontaneous voluntary actions are preceded by a readiness potential starting some 550 msecs before the act. If the act is less spontaneous, the potential appears 800 msecs or more beforehand. With characteristic ingenuity, Libet got people to say when they became aware of an intention to act (by getting them to relate the onset of their awareness to the position of a 'clock' hand as it moved round a dial). He found that the readiness potential always began about 350 msecs *before* awareness of any intention to act. In other words, initiation of voluntary actions happens quite unconsciously – our feeling that consciousness is directly responsible is an illusion. Of course, awareness still appears before the act is carried out, except in the case of very fast responses which we in fact usually recognise as having been 'reflex' or 'automatic'. With so-called 'voluntary' acts, there is still a time window of 150 – 200 msecs in which awareness might give a final veto or go-ahead to the action.

Here are some of Libet's (1993) comments about his work:

Many, if not most, mental functions or events proceed without any reportable awareness . . . even complex functions, as in problem-solving or intuitive and creative thinking. On the other hand, the simplest kinds of mental functions can be accompanied by awareness/subjective experience, like awareness of a tap on the skin . . . It is not, then, simply the complexity or creativeness of a mental function that imparts to it the quality of subjective awareness of what is going on. The cerebral code for the distinction between the appearance or absence of awareness in any mental operation would seem to require a mediating neuronal mechanism uniquely related to awareness *per se* rather than to complexity, etc.

He goes on to say that neuronal activities become conscious only if they persist for sufficiently long, even though briefer activity is perfectly adequate for information processing and making coherent responses. However, although he points out that '. . . awareness of an event [does] not appear at the onset of an appropriate series of neural activities and develop gradually. Conscious experience of events, whether initiated exogenously or endogenously, [has] a unitary discontinuous quality', he was not able to identify any particular neuronal events (other than duration) associated with the sudden appearance of awareness.

The findings concerning 'voluntary' actions have obvious but important implications for ideas about free will, which is a topic that we shall save up for Chapter 6. Libet concludes that they constrain its operation to a very late phase in the development of action. However, there is also an earlier phase in which it may act that he does not mention in the paper from which the quotations were taken (he has done so elsewhere), namely the choice of the range of potential actions. If his subjects had chosen not to participate in his experiments, they would have had a different set of readiness potentials from the ones that he measured. This might be thought too obvious to be worth mentioning, but his findings are so impressive that admiration for discoveries about the tactical constraints on awareness can easily cause one to lose sight of the broader, strategic role that it may have.

Does one have to accept these findings at face value? Eccles (1985) has pointed out that the ones concerning voluntary actions can be reconciled with his own view of consciousness which is dualistic in the Cartesian tradition. He proposes an immaterial consciousness which can alter the probability of neurotransmitter release and has learned to time its actions to coincide with favourable spontaneous fluctuations of that probability. This seems to account all right for the Libet findings, though it multiplies entities in a way that William of Occam (the originator of Occam's razor) might not have liked.

A simpler proposal is that the time delays are needed, not for awareness to occur, but for the ability to report on an awareness to develop. It's the familiar problem about distinguishing awareness from the capacity to remember it cropping up yet again. In this context it is especially perplexing as the whole tenor of Libet's work suggests that awareness and reverberating, short-term memory are closely inter-linked. Two bits of evidence are rather against any simple 'ability to report' account; first, the difference in subjective timing between experiences due to stimulation outside and inside the brain; second, the fact that the quality of an experience due to outside stimulation can be altered by later cortical stimulation. The first would require one to envisage some sort of systematic distortion of reportage according to source of stimulus, which is not that strong an objection as Libet proposed something very similar in relation to awareness. The second poses greater difficulties, however. One could account for it using, for instance, Dennett's (1991) 'multiple draft' model of consciousness which says that it emerges from layered patterns of brief memories subject to constant revision. The catch is that the second stimulus does not appear to be subject to the same time constraints as the first in relation to reporting on it. Why not? This does not pose a problem for Libet's own interpretation of his findings since awareness can presumably be modified by any relevant happening prior to its sudden crystallisation; a memory, however, is a different matter. It should either be fixed once and for all or later events should require as long to achieve reportability as earlier ones, and this is not what seems to occur. Though one must have doubts, Libet's interpretation of his work seems a lot better than alternatives.

CONCLUSIONS

Three themes have dominated this Chapter. The first is that, despite a subjective feeling of smooth continuity, awareness is 'chunked' with respect to time. Perhaps this is not so surprising when one remembers that there are minimum spatio-temporal units of information in the brain (the individual depolarisation waves spreading over nerve cell membranes). What is surprising is that chunks of awareness are so long. There is general agreement that the minimum perceptual duration, i.e. the shortest chunk, for conscious perception is around 100 msecs the clock timing it probably being one or more of the alpha rhythms. It's not really known whether the other EEG rhythms also mark subdivisions of awareness in relation to time. If they don't, one can think of the flow of consciousness as being a little like a cine film where the rapid succession of still pictures gives an illusion of smooth flow. It isn't very like a cine film, though, as each 'still' also contains a picture of the temporal relationships of the items within it.

Then there is the realisation that functional units in the brain are defined, not only by their spatial relationships and interconnections, but also by ever-shifting patterns of coherent, synchronised, rhythmic electrical activity. These spatio-temporally defined patterns of activity certainly underpin awareness, but they develop within a few milliseconds and must therefore (so Libet's findings imply) also underpin unconscious mental functions. It's not known whether patterns associated with awareness have any special characteristics, though the indications are that there is nothing startlingly different about them since anything obvious would probably have been noticed.

Finally, there is Libet whose work shows conclusively that we always live up to half a second behind the times, if one follows the usual assumption that 'we' consist of our awareness. Perhaps of greater importance from the point of view of understanding consciousness is his conclusion that the development of awareness is the result of a process taking around 300 to 500 msecs, though awareness itself occurs as a discontinuity, a sudden happening analogous to crystallisation or precipitation. It's not absolutely certain that the findings must be interpreted like this, but there's not all that much room for doubt. The main casualty of accepting the obvious interpretation is any hope that coherent EEG activity on its own can account for the binding problem in relation to awareness since epochs of coherent activity are reaching their end before awareness occurs.

Given that so much about our experience of time is illusory, it is not surprising that we have no good vocabulary with which to describe it. The words that we use are shadows of shadows. 'Now' refers to my automatic referral backward in time of my current experience to the first arrival of information concerning it. 'Wait a moment!' really ought to be accompanied by a specification of how aroused I am since the moment, depending on my internal state, could be anything from 100 msecs to 10 seconds by clock time. 'I'm doing this as quickly as possible' means that my brain has already prepared the action and is simply waiting for my laggard consciousness to give it the go-ahead, perhaps, or perhaps consciousness is simply watching what is going ahead anyway and the 'I' should refer not to my awareness as I assume, but simply to a chunk of neural activity involving my motor cortex among other areas.

Our butterfly awareness is clearly a creature that likes to mimic the life cycle of the insect species. Not only does it flit from part to part of the brain quilt but, having settled on a particular patch, it has to pupate for quite a while before reappearing in its full glory. Though it may be a product of brain activity, it seems to live in a different conceptual world from neurotransmitters or depolarisation waves.

REFERENCES

Barinaga, M. (1990) 'The Mind Revealed?', *Science* 249, 856–8.
Basar, E. (1992) 'Brain Natural Frequencies are Causal Factors for Resonances and Induced Rhythms', in *Induced Rhythms in the Brain*, E. Basar and T.H. Bullock (eds), Birkhauser: Boston.
Basar-Eroglu, C., Basar, E., Demiralp, T. and Schurmann, M. (1992) 'P300–Response: Possible Psychophysiological Correlates in Delta and Theta Frequency Channels. A Review', *International Journal of Psychophysiology* 13, 161–79.
Bressler, S.L., Coppola, R. and Nakamura, R. (1993) 'Episodic Multiregional Cortical Coherence at Multiple Frequencies During Visual Task Performance', *Nature* 366, 153–6.
Brown, J.W. (1990) 'Psychology of Time Awareness', *Brain and Cognition* 14, 144–64.
Cook, J.E. (1991) 'Correlated Activity in the CNS: A Role on Every Timescale?', *Trends in Neurosciences* 14, 397–401.
Dennett, D.C. (1991) *Consciousness Explained*, Penguin Books: Harmondsworth.
Eccles, J.C. (1985) 'Mental Summation: The Timing of Voluntary Intentions by Cortical Activity', *Behavioural and Brain Sciences* 8 (4), 542–3.
Gerstner, W., Ritz, R. and van Hemmen, J.L. (1993) 'Why Spikes? Hebbian Learning and Retrieval of Time-Resolved Excitation Patterns', *Biological Cybernetics* 69, 503–15.
Libet, B. (1989) 'Conscious Subjective Experience vs. Unconscious Mental Functions: A Theory of the Cerebral Processes Involved', in *Models of Brain Function*, R. Cotterill (ed.), Cambridge University Press.
—— (1993) 'The Neural Time Factor in Conscious and Unconscious Events', in *Experimental and Theoretical Studies of Consciousness*, CIBA Foundation Symposium 174, Wiley: Chichester.
Lockwood, M. (1989) *Mind, Brain and the Quantum*, Basil Blackwell: Oxford.
Nunn, C.M.H. (1980) 'A Model of the Functional Psychoses', *Acta Psychiatrica Scandinavica* 75–84.
Nunn, C.M.H. and Osselton, J.W. (1974) 'The Influence of the EEG Alpha Rhythm on the Perception of Visual Stimuli', *Psychophysiology* 11, 294–303.
Ray, W.J. and Cole, H.W. (1985) 'EEG Alpha Activity Reflects Attentional Demands, and Beta Activity Reflects Emotional and Cognitive Processes', *Science* 228, 750–52.
Salmelin, R., Hari, R., Lounasmaa, O.V. and Sams, M. (1994) 'Dynamics of Brain Activation During Picture Naming', *Nature* 368, 463–5.
Whitehead, A.N. (1978 edn) *Process and Reality*, Free Press: New York.

3 The nature of matter

It has become ever more clear over the past 70 years that reality is best described by a theory that no one fully understands and which cannot be applied to most everyday phenomena. Quantum theory has been subjected to many stringent tests and all of its predictions, however strange, have *always* been borne out. Originally developed to account for why atoms do not collapse and why they radiate and absorb energy in discrete amounts (quanta), it has now gone far beyond these rather simple beginnings. It is essentially a mathematical theory, so trying to describe it in words is analogous to transforming a picture into a poem. Inaccuracies, distortions and over-simplifications inevitably creep in. Nevertheless, one can convey the essence of the picture, and that is what is attempted here. Some grasp of what the material world is really like, and of the unfamiliar ways in which it can behave, is probably necessary to reaching an understanding of awareness and is certainly needed to comprehend the experimental evidence set out in Chapter 5.

Quantum theory gives two alternative pictures of the nature of a particle of matter which are in fact mathematically equivalent. One is of a line travelling through a wavery, multi-dimensional space (the Heisenberg picture); the other is of a wave of possibilities or potentialities evolving with time in normal, three-dimensional space (the Schrodinger picture). Every so often something entirely different happens; the Heisenberg line reduces to a point, or the Schrodinger wave function collapses, and a manifestation occurs in our everyday physical world. The type of manifestation observed is partly dependent on the nature of the apparatus used to observe it. If you are looking for wave energy that is what you will observe; if you are looking for where a particle is situated, you will find one somewhere. If you try looking for both at the same time, you are welcome to do so but one of them will be a bit 'fuzzy' – or very fuzzy indeed if your measurement of the other 'observable' is very precise. This is the famous Heisenberg uncertainty principle.

Most people find it easier to handle the Schrodinger picture, because it retains a concept of ordinary 3D space, so we shall stick with that one here. The wave function actually consists of a range of probability amplitudes relating to the various potentialities that exist (i.e. position in space, momentum, spin angle, etc.). When it collapses a potentiality compatible with the observational apparatus will become manifest, but it is impossible to predict which of the compatible alternatives will appear; manifestation occurs at random, the probability of any particular observation being related to its amplitude in the wave function.

The reason that quantum theory is mostly confined to describing very small entities is that the mathematics of the wave function are complicated, and complications increase at an exponential rate as the number of interacting quantum objects increases. The equations for three such interacting objects already present impossible difficulties. All the same, not all single quantum objects are small. It is thought that neutron stars, for instance, can be described by the equations for a single entity, but weigh considerably more than the sun.

COMPLEX NUMBERS

The numbers used to specify the wave function are worth describing as they give a flavour of the whole concept of reality that may be needed to get to grips with awareness. They are called 'complex' as they have two components; first, an ordinary real number of the sort that we all use every day – 1, 2, 3, etc.; second, an imaginary number.

Of course all numbers are in a sense imaginary, and the so-called 'imaginary' ones are no more artificial than the 'real' ones. What they are is a set of numbers – 1, 2, 3, etc. – that have no connection whatsoever with the set that we use for everyday purposes. They can be pictured as existing on a different dimension that is at right angles to the dimension on which everyday numbers exist.

'Imaginary' numbers are specified by taking a 'real' number and multiplying it by the square root of minus 1. This is something that cannot exist in the world of 'real' numbers. It's a sort of one phrase mathematical impossibility, so it is good for defining a set of numbers utterly different from the 'real' set. It has another interesting property; namely that, when squared, it becomes minus 1 so in effect disappearing. When you square an 'imaginary' number you get a 'real' one.

This mathematical picture seems to be telling us that there is a component of the wave function which is totally unrelated to our ordinary systems of measurement, and perhaps even to our everyday world. Squaring the wave function converts the probability amplitudes into an ordinary probability that can be handled with everyday statistics. This is the mathematical operation that corresponds with collapse of the wave function when an observation is made.

One may be tempted to think that all this is just playing with symbols and that neither complex numbers nor the wave function have any existence outside the heads of mathematicians; they are just useful concepts for calculating certain esoteric results. This was in effect the view taken by Niels Bohr who did more than anyone else to nurture the growth of quantum physics in the period between the two World Wars. However, as we shall see later, it is not a correct view. The wave function is nearly as real as anything else that passes for reality, and the implications of complex numbers have to be taken seriously.

COLLAPSE OF THE WAVE FUNCTION

Before the wave function collapses, all the potentialities in it coexist in what is termed 'superposition'. This causes a problem as any interacting system, says quantum theory, has to be considered a whole in a very profound sense. You cannot say that the idea of superposition need apply only to the sub-atomic particles in an object, or that one part of a system can be in superposition while another is permanently collapsed.

In what was probably at the time a whimsical spirit, intended to show up the absurdities of the quantum view of things, Schrodinger pictured his famous but unfortunate cat. This poor beast was in a box with an ampoule of deadly gas and an apparatus designed to release the gas if a single radioactive atom should decay. The box was to be opened when the chance that the atom would have decayed was exactly even. According to quantum theory, immediately before the lid was lifted, the wave function of the atom would have equal amplitudes for decay and non-decay, observing it would collapse the wave function and one or other possibility would be manifest. One can live with this as a picture of the atom's state, but the trouble is that exactly the same considerations ought to apply to the cat. When looked at it will be found to be either alive or dead, but immediately before this it must have been in a superposition of both states; it was not even half-alive and half-dead, it was both wholly alive *and* wholly dead. An absurd picture indeed, but one that won't go away. There are technical difficulties about applying the idea of the Schrodinger wave function to entities like cats in thermal equilibrium with the environment; the related notion of a quantum 'density matrix' is more appropriate. However, we shall stick with the cat metaphor since it is so vivid and has such a long history. Quantum theory is correct, so all the tests tell us; therefore, some way has to be found to accommodate the superimposed cat. Ideas about what is going on when collapse happens offer various ways of doing this.

There are basically three explanations:

1 The paradox is real, but there is no point in worrying about it. Collapse occurs as a consequence of observation and you can never know what really happened before it, even if the wave function is anything more than a convenient abstraction for calculating the outcome of observations like the one just made on our poor cat.
2 The wave function does not collapse. What really happens is that reality divides so that there is a world with a live cat in it and another with a dead cat. Both the possible outcomes will be observed somewhere.
3 Collapse of the wave function is caused, not by observation, but by some physical circumstance or process which ensures that the cat would have been either alive or dead at the relevant time even if the box had remained closed. States such as a superposition of a live and a dead cat occur so briefly that they do not intrude on the real world.

Answer 1, though the prevalent view among physicists at least up to a decade or so ago, is a bit of a cop out and not worth dwelling on. To accept it is to give up on a fascinating area of enquiry. There is a variant of it, due originally to De Broglie, which says that particles are particles but they are accompanied by an immaterial wave (called a 'pilot wave') which is nevertheless material enough to affect their trajectories. This idea has gone on cropping up for about sixty years, but has never found much general favour. On it, the cat would be wholly alive until it was wholly dead but there would also be a ghostly cat existing in superposition until the box was opened. It implies a very different view of reality from the standard Heisenberg or Schrodinger one which has a certain 'naturalistic' appeal when thinking about the wave/particle duality, but actually makes it a lot more difficult to envisage other important variables such as spin.

Answer 2 comes in two main varieties. First, there is the relative state formulation of Everett, better known as the 'Many Worlds Theory'. This monstrous edifice holds that, when the box is opened, the observer and the whole universe divide into two. In one universe the observer sees a dead cat and in the other a live one. Of course, the same thing has to be regarded as happening every time any wave function appears to collapse anywhere. Countless billions of universes spawned every second; nature may be profligate but this seems ridiculous. The theory does have two virtues: it avoids many of the puzzles associated with the idea of collapse; it also provides a natural explanation in mathematical terms for why the wave function has to be squared to get from probability amplitudes to classical probabilities. The game, however, seems hardly worth the candle. People have tried to reduce the costs by saying that most universes will be so similar that you could not tell the difference, or that it is only the observer that divides (many biographies instead of many worlds). Papering over the cracks in this way seems hardly worth while because the theory could never be tested (see Note). Whatever experimental results you got in a test, you could always say that you just happened to be living in some (improbable) branch of the universe that fitted them.

The other type 2 answer is due to Bohm (1983). He proposed that the wave function and all its manifestations is itself a manifestation of a sub-quantum reality that he termed the 'holomovement'. The idea seems to be that the holomovement evolves throwing up manifestations, including us the observers, that we perceive as real and then sucking them back into its own true reality. Thus, the cat might be really dead in our semi-illusory world, but there is also a live cat plus an observer viewing it tucked away as a potentiality elsewhere in the holomovement. This idea has a certain beauty, and may for all we know be true, but seems more mystical than scientific. A more advanced science might be able to handle it but we need sharper, less global hypotheses at present.

This leaves answers in category 3 of which there are three to describe at present. They seem so obviously on the right lines that one can expect that a range of competitors of this type will soon be battling it out and then we shall know what causes collapse of the wave function, if indeed there is only one cause; perhaps several different mechanisms can cause collapse. The first to be described was the GRW theory (so-called due to Ghirardi, Rimini and Weber, 1986). This says that very occasionally the wave functions of particles collapse spontaneously into one of the positional possibilities for that particle. This happens so infrequently to any individual particle that it has never been noticed in experiments on single particles. However, when you have a mass of associated particles comprising a cat or a house or whatever, there are so many that one at least will be collapsed at any given moment, so keeping its associates localised too. Hence, you never get more than the most fleeting superposition when dealing with something so large as a cat. It seems a good theory except that there is no obvious reason why wave functions should collapse by themselves in the required manner. It is unproven.

Next, the Penrose hypothesis, which is more interesting as it gives a role to gravity. One of the great goals of present-day physics is to reconcile quantum theory with general relativity. These two have always been at odds even though Einstein made major contributions to the first as well as originating the second. There are hypothetical quantum particles of gravity called gravitons. Efforts are at present being made to detect them by a number of laboratories. What Penrose's theory said was that the wave function collapses in the familiar random way when one possibility in it acquires a mass difference from the other possibilities of more than one graviton. He has modified the idea a bit since first proposing it. His latest suggestion is that it's not all or nothing due to a one graviton difference; rather, the *rate* of collapse depends on the size of gravitational energy differences between different possibilities in superposition. Collapse will take a very long time for anything as small as an isolated nuclear particle, but will be very fast for objects as big as a speck of dust, say. It's a plausible idea as the presence of a gravitational difference implies a bending of space; maybe the wave function cannot cope if one of its components gets bent relative to the others. Collapse will not happen (or in the latest version will take millions of years to happen) with individual particles if they are on their own, but as soon as they come to interact with observers or with each other in things like cats then the wave function of the entire particle/observer system or that of the radioactive atom/cat will readily show large gravitational energy differences. A live cat, for instance, will be breathing, pumping blood, etc., all of which will make for weighty differences from its dead counterpart. Therefore, superpositions of live and dead cats will collapse so fast that you never catch a whisker of them. I've spelled this theory out in a little more detail than the others both for its intrinsic interest and because a grasp of its outlines is important to understanding an experiment that will be described in Chapter 5.

Third, is Marshall's very recent theory which I may well not have understood correctly. He seems to be saying that collapse happens when its occurrence will favour the manifestation of certain sorts of phase coherence, particularly the sorts that occur in highly ordered structures like crystals or may, he believes, exist in very complicated ones like living organisms. If this is his meaning, the theory should be easy to test as all that would be necessary would be to remove the cat from the box in some experiments and to look to see whether the ampoule of poison gas was intact instead of looking to see whether the cat was dead. On

Marshall's theory you would have to wait somewhat longer to have an exactly even chance of finding a dead cat than to have the same chance of finding a smashed ampoule when the cat was absent. The actual experiment, of course, could be done with bacteria or possibly different types of inanimate set-up. There would be absolutely no need to really kill any cats which is only proposed for its vividness and long history as a thought experiment. As theories are valuable in proportion, among other things, to their testability, this may well be the most useful of all the collapse theories provided it does not turn out to contradict what is already known about the randomness of collapse.

It's worth a reminder at this stage that the ideas set out above really apply only to classes of objects which are not particularly like cats (they must be very small, very cold or very coherent). With objects as big, hot and inchoate as cats, Schrodinger's mathematics show that thermal (heat) interactions with their environment will cause decoherence of the quantum density matrix which is a related idea to wave function collapse (see Zurek, 1991). This seems at first sight to provide a nice naturalistic account which leaves one freed from all worry about the possibility of ghostly quantum superpositions being relevant in our everyday world. Unfortunately, quantum objects do exist in the everyday world (e.g. the laser light which enables your CD player to work). It has been pointed out (by Penrose) that observations of a quantum object which *fail to detect it*, so that the object apparently had no interaction with the rest of the world, nevertheless affect the object's state in a manner which can later be shown to have consequences for the real world (see Penrose, 1994: 259–86). Also, there's no reason why one outcome rather than another should be favoured when the matrix decoheres – which raises the 'Many Worlds' spectre once again! Although many people would like to pretend that superpositions are just a mathematical convenience, they are either far more than that or else our everyday so-called 'reality' is no more than a mathematical construct.

HOW REAL IS THE WAVE FUNCTION?

Just as individual particles and assemblies of particles are each thought to have their unique wave function, so also the entire universe has its wave function albeit a rather complicated one! This means that there is a wave function occupying the whole of space and time, including the apparently empty vacuum of space. If it has any reality it should have effects, which indeed turns out to be the case. There are major mathematical problems in quantum theory due to the fact that, when you try to calculate the energy associated with a single point in space, the answer comes out 'it is infinite'. This is probably because a point is dimensionless while there may be a minimum quantum unit of length (and hence volume) just as there is a minimum unit of energy. All the same, the potential energy content of empty space is arbitrarily high.

The current picture of the vacuum is of a sort of frothing sea of particles and energy, sparkling in and out of existence so fast that energy conservation laws are not broken. Danah Zohar has written a rather beautiful Chapter in her recent book (Zohar and Marshall, 1993) comparing the modern idea of the vacuum to the Buddhist concept of the void, replete with all potentiality. We and our whole world can be thought of as simply ripples on its surface. More prosaically, quantum chromodynamics (the theory describing the atomic nucleus and the forces which hold it together) tells us that these evanescent, 'virtual' particles that flash from the void and disappear play an essential part in keeping nuclei together. It is tautologous, but nevertheless true, to say that if the wave function of the universe was not real neither would we exist. There's been a fascinating suggestion recently (Matthews, 1994) that one of the most familiar and irritating of all phenomena to mobile creatures like us, inertia, is due to virtual particles in the vacuum putting up a resistance to us accelerating the particles of our own bodies past them.

There is a more straightforward reason for thinking that all the components of a superposition have a real existence and are not just mathematical abstractions. They have actually been 'seen', it is claimed (by Clark, 1991), albeit under a very special set of circumstances. As we shall see later, the electrical current in a superconductor can be considered to be a single quantum object. If you make a super-conductor into a ring with a very narrow bit in one place, you get a device called a SQUID (Superconducting Quantum Interference Device) in which the electromagnetic flux can occur with a number of discrete values which may exist in superposition. Clark was able, in effect, to detect two of the discrete values at the same time. In other words, he may have shown that the different parts of a superposition can be detected *before* collapse of the wave function.

Clark himself suggested that he was able to detect its components without causing collapse of the wave function because the quantum object that he studied (the electromagnetic flux in the SQUID) was actually larger than the detection apparatus, which fitted inside the ring. However, it seems difficult to reconcile his finding with collapse accounts of type 1. More important, from our point of view, is the fact that the finding makes it easier to think of real processes that might have meaningful outcomes occurring in the pre-collapse realm.

NON-LOCALITY

Quantum theory has a curious way of dealing with space, even though position in space is a very important 'quantum observable'. For some purposes space is a precisely defined circumstance, but there are other conditions in which it appears partly or wholly irrelevant. There seems to be a strong indication that space is not such a fundamental quality as it appears to us in our everyday world, or for that matter as it is taken to be (in the form of space-time) in general relativity.

For instance, an electron forming part of an electric current will suddenly come to occupy a volume thousands of times greater than the moment before if the current goes superconducting. This is not a very good example because it is not strictly speaking meaningful to talk of an individual electron in a superconducting current. However, there is a much weirder result that has attracted enormous interest since Einstein called attention to it, in much the same spirit as Schrodinger to his cat, as an example of the absurdity of quantum theory.

What Einstein and two associates pointed out was that quantum theory implies that, if two particles have at any time been associated (in certain precisely defined senses of the word), then observing some feature of one of them will instantaneously determine the outcome of a similar observation on the other even if it is now on the opposite side of the galaxy. It is as if there is no space between them, however far apart they appear to us. For a long time this paradox was treated as a curiosity only, but then John Bell reformulated it and showed how it could be tested. The crucial experiments were done by a team in Paris led by Alain Aspect. The chances are that particles do actually behave in these circumstances as if spatial separation did not matter or did not exist. Although of great theoretical interest, this phenomenon could not be put to practical use in a communication device since there is no way in which it could be used to transmit information. It does not really undermine general relativity.

It appears that there is a way of escaping the 'non-locality' conclusion, which was suggested by Feynman (1991), namely to assume that negative probabilities exist. If you try to think of what a negative probability could be you quickly get dizzy, but maybe they can be thought of like imaginary numbers as convenient mathematical abstractions. However, we have already seen that imaginary numbers are more than this; they are a symbol for some uncomfortable aspect of reality. It is not clear that what a negative probability might be a symbol for would be any more congenial than having to think of space as some sort of secondary, derivative property. Scully *et al.* (1994), in a paper too technical to describe in detail here, recently discussed Feynman's idea and concluded that it does simplify the spatial conceptual problems associated with quantum theory, but there is an implication that this was at the expense of increasing the difficulty of conceiving temporal linkages between particles.

BOSE–EINSTEIN CONDENSATES

Particles can be classified in all sorts of ways. A particularly important division is into fermions (after the Italian physicist Fermi) and bosons (after the Indian physicist Bose). Fermions obey the Pauli exclusion principle which says that no two such particles can occupy the same quantum state at the same time. Electrons are fermions which is just as well because it is the Pauli principle which stops atoms from collapsing in on themselves. Bosons behave the opposite way; given half a chance they will occupy the same state forming a unity in which it is not meaningful to talk of separate particles. Photons (the particle aspects of electromagnetic radiation) are like this. So, interestingly enough, are electron pairs. This is because fermions have ½ spin and bosons 0, 1 or 2 spins; hence two fermions can in appropriate circumstances make a boson. It is a good illustration of the fact that the wave function of associated particles may have radically different properties from the functions of the same particles when separate. It's also a finding which cannot be reconciled with any simple version of De Broglie's pilot wave idea, the main appeal of which lay in apparent, but as it turns out delusory, naturalism.

The process of forming this unity is termed Bose–Einstein condensation. It is a bit like what happens when an orchestra stops tuning up and starts playing. Suddenly the cacophony vanishes and all the strings, say, start producing a recognisably single harmony. Of course, the only way that violins can do this is through the skill of their players, but if the energy supply rate from the bows to the strings were enormously greater than is in fact possible, they could come to vibrate in harmony automatically through condensation among the quantum particles corresponding to vibrational energy (phonons).

Bose–Einstein condensates are thus describable by the wave function equations for single quantum objects, but are nevertheless quite large. They can extend over inches or even further. The best known examples are laser activity, superconductivity and superfluidity. The latter two occur only in extremely cold materials as they are fragile and can be readily disrupted by the thermal motion of molecules. Laser activity is robust, however, and can occur at very high temperatures. The condensations which may occur between more exotic particles such as phonons are likely also to be fairly robust. This opens up the interesting possibility that some of them might happen in biological systems (see Chapter 1, 'exotica' and 'conclusions').

TIME IN QUANTUM THEORY

This is where the theory starts running into major problems. The wave function evolves smoothly and deterministically through time, interrupted by the discontinuities introduced by episodic collapse, but there is no reason why it should go in one direction rather than another; it could just as well run backwards as far as the equations are concerned. Moreover, position in time, unlike position in space, is not used as a quantum observable. There is Richard Feynman's well-known idea that there may be only one particle of each type existing in space-time as an incredibly tangled ball of string and appearing to us as separate particles wherever it crosses the 'plane' of the present in three-dimensional space. However, the idea does not account for the existence of the present or for why it should appear to us to move so steadily and inexorably onwards.

People usually invoke the second law of thermodynamics to explain the direction that time takes; the one that says that on average entropy (a measure of disorder) increases. The picture is of time being heaved along by a sort of irreversible ratchet because 'all quantum measurements to date are thermodynamically irreversible' (Percival, 1991). It is not clear, however, that this statement is quite accurate; the formation of a Bose–Einstein condensate, for example, might fit at least some of the criteria for a quantum measurement but is accompanied by a local *decrease* in entropy.

Penrose says that the arrow of time was built in right from the beginning as the big bang in which the universe was formed had an extremely low entropy while black holes, into which bits of the universe are disappearing piecemeal, have an extremely high entropy. This seems at first sight to be wrong as the universe at the time of the big bang is thought to have been in thermal equilibrium (i.e. had very high entropy), while recent studies of the cosmic background radiation (Turner, 1993) show that at only a few hundred thousand years old (present age about 15 billion years) it fairly definitely had high entropy. However, Penrose (1986) distinguishes between entropy of gravitational and of thermal origin; the former was allegedly extremely small at the time of the big bang and outweighed the influence of the latter. All the same, we don't yet seem to have any wholly consistent explanation of why time goes one way rather than another, let alone of why there should be a present moment.

Perhaps something can be made of the fact that there are sub-atomic processes, involving the weak nuclear force, which are *not* symmetrical with regard to time; that is, they behave differently when the equations are run forward through time than when the maths is done backwards (Landsberg 1982). Theorists have not been very excited about this because temporal symmetry is thought to be preserved when additional variables are also taken into account (charge and parity). But maybe one could argue on this basis that the direction time takes has something to do with the fact that more matter than anti-matter was produced in the big bang at the beginning of the universe. Because it's possible to regard anti-matter particles as ordinary ones that happen to be running backwards in time, and because there are few anti-particles around, maybe time for us will on average appear to go in only one direction. It's a field where ideas are aplenty but consensus absent.

If time were a quantum observable, it would probably commute with energy in the same way that position commutes with momentum – i.e. you can measure one or other exactly but not both together. This is implicit in the picture of the vacuum allowing the appearance of highly energetic particles from nowhere provided they exist for only very short periods. The other side of this coin, of course, is that, if the energy of a particle were exactly measured, its time would become completely indeterminate. One can have fun trying to picture what the concept of an indeterminate time might mean in this context.

Lockwood (1989: 284) suggested that the relationship between the past moments and the present moment of any individual consciousness might be one of linear superposition. Although an attractive concept, it may soon be proved untenable at least in such a simple form, as it appears that there is a temporal version of Bell's inequality (the theory which encouraged Alain Aspect and his team to show that one measurement can determine the outcome of another regardless of spatial separation). This time-related version suggests that, between measurement events, particular histories are not an element of reality because all possible histories of a quantum particle exist in super-position (Gribbin, 1993). If all possible histories exist in superposition, it is hard to see how a succession of particular past moments could do so as well (see Laszlo, 1993: Chapter 8, for a non-mathematical, speculative account of how 'memories' of any sort might be imprinted on the vacuum). The relevant experiment has not been done yet, so the issue is still in doubt.

If experiment should show past time to contain a *mélange* of all possible histories, there may still be one circumstance in which Lockwood's speculation could continue to be entertained; that is if awareness consists of a succession of Bose condensates each with a unique topology. Such condensates are single quantum objects and, if unique, might be able to retain this quality in relation to other such entities in a historical superposition. Of course, immediately before each condensate formed, there would have been several alternatives in superposition so a lot hangs on whether uniqueness of shape might be able to retrospectively exclude other possibilities from any hypothetical historical superposition of an individual person's awarenesses. Perhaps it may one day be possible to formulate ideas of this type in a sufficiently coherent way to allow conclusions to be drawn, especially as the notion of backward causation has philosophical respectability (Dummett, 1986). However, the whole topic is very obscure at present.

One of the most dramatic events known to psychiatrists is the extraordinary vividness with which people can sometimes relive a traumatic event which may have occurred half a lifetime or more ago. Anyone who has witnessed, or experienced, such a reliving must have doubts about whether it could be based solely on the reactivation of old neural engrams. Maybe the nature of reality allows direct access to the experience itself. For the time being at least, theory does not rule out such a possibility.

CONCLUSIONS

Although quantum theory is very strange, it is not in fact particularly mysterious. There are mysteries to be sure, to do with time, why particles and forces should be as they are and how general relativity fits into the picture, but these lie outside present-day quantum theory. Non-specialists wanting a brief, clear account of the strangeness and the limitations of present-day physics can find a good one in Chapters 2, 3 and 4 of Laszlo's (1993) book. It is as accurate as possible for a short description that contains no mathematics, despite the inaccuracies in his subsequent account of neo-Darwinism which is marred by too frequent use of what has been called 'the argument from personal incredulity'.

Most people will remember the shock that they got as schoolchildren when they first learned that a table, for instance, is made up of atoms and, contrary to all appearances, consists mostly of empty space. The quantum view of reality is truer than the atomic view, even though it does not yet give a complete account of the physical world, but most of us come to it when we are already adult and cannot so easily accommodate a totally new way of looking at things. It can appear mysterious but only because it conflicts with our in-built cognitive structures (to put it kindly) or obstinate prejudices (to be more direct).

To use the concepts of quantum theory in relation to trying to account for awareness is clearly *not* to try to explain one mystery in terms of another, as critics have claimed. Rather, it is to try to explain a subtle and mysterious phenomenon (awareness) in terms of the most reliable picture of the nature of the world that we have. Some of the theories outlined in the next Chapter have gone a surprising distance towards achieving that aim.

NOTE

Deutsch (1986) speculated that one might in principle be able to tell the difference between the Everett world view and others by looking at interference effects in artificial memories. However, a positive result from any such experiment would be open to many interpretations, while a negative one could not falsify the 'many worlds' view for the reason given above – i.e. there would be no way of proving that you did not just happen to be living in a strange world which chanced to give your particular set of results.

REFERENCES

Bohm, D. (1983) *Wholeness and the Implicate Order*, Ark: London.

Clark, T.D. (1991) 'Macroscopic Quantum Objects', in *Quantum Implications*, B.J. Hiley and F.D. Peat (eds), Routledge: London.

Deutsch, D. (1986) Reported in *The Ghost in the Atom*, P.C.W. Davies and J.R. Brown (eds), Cambridge University Press.

Dummett, M. (1986) 'Causal Loops', in *The Nature of Time*, R. Flood and M. Lockwood (eds), Basil Blackwell: Oxford.

Feynman, R.P. (1991) 'Negative Probability', in *Quantum Implications*, B.J. Hiley and F.D. Peat (eds), Routledge: London.

Ghirardi, G.C., Rimini, A. and Weber, T. (1986) 'Unified Dynamics for Microscopic and Macroscopic Systems', *American Physical Society Review* 34 (2), 470–91.

Gribbin, J. (1993) 'Do Electrons Have a Past?', *New Scientist*, 4 December, 14–15.

Landsberg, P.T. (1982) *Introduction: The Enigma of Time*, Adam Hilger: Bristol.

Laszlo, E. (1993) *The Creative Cosmos*, Floris Books: Edinburgh.

Lockwood, M. (1989) *Mind, Brain and the Quantum: The Compound I*, Basil Blackwell: Oxford.

Marshall, I.N. (1993) *A Unified Dynamics of Consciousness and Quantum Collapse* (to be published).

Matthews, R. (1994) 'Inertia: Does Empty Space Put up Resistance?', *Science*, 263, 612–13.

Penrose, R. (1986) 'Big Bangs, Black Holes and "Time's Arrow",' in *The Nature of Time*, R. Flood and M. Lockwood (eds), Basil Blackwell Oxford.

—— (1989) *The Emperor's New Mind*, Oxford University Press.

—— (1994) *Shadows of the Mind*, Oxford University Press.

Percival, I. (1991) 'Quantum Measurement Theory and Experiment', in *Macroscopic Quantum Phenomena*, T.D. Clark, H. Prance, T. Spiller (eds), World Scientific.

Scully, M.O., Walther, H. and Schleich, W. (1994) 'Feynman's Approach to Negative Probability in Quantum Mechanics', *Physical Review A*. 49 (3), 1562–6.

Turner, M.S. (1993) 'Why is the Temperature of the Universe 2.276Kelvin?', *Science* 262, 861–6.

Zohar, D. and Marshall, I. (1993) *The Quantum Society*, Bloomsbury: London.

Zurek, W.H. (1991) 'Decoherence and the Transition from Quantum to Classical', *Physics Today*, October, 36–44.

4 Various theories

'Consciousness is elusive, and trying to think about it can make you unhappy', wrote Honderich (1987). Being a philosopher, ideas should not have made him unhappy and perhaps the 'you' in the quotation was significant. Certainly, he went on to describe with much gusto contemporary confusion over how to think about mind/brain relationships, coming up with the conclusion that the idea he likes is that of a 'nomic' connection between the two. This apparently means a law-like relationship that falls somewhere between identity and independence.

However, all possible ideas about the way in which mind and brain are connected have their advocates even if some are less fashionable than others, some on the way up and others going down. It's the uncertainty and the endless space for theorising that make for unhappiness. One longs, after a time, for a solid stone to kick in the manner of Dr Johnson when he refuted idealism (the philosophy which holds that things don't exist independently of awareness of them). There are stones, even though they are not that solidly grounded, but they have been herded, to mix metaphors, into the next Chapter. Readers who become sickened by too much theory are welcome to skip on to it, but please pause at the sections on Penrose and on Marshall, as well as at the 'conclusions', or an important part of the next Chapter will be unintelligible.

The current range of ideas has been set out in detail by Jean Burns (1990), and makes a long and involved list with many loops and subtleties of distinction. The range extends from identity theories, that mind is simply the result of complex electrochemical processes in the brain, to the belief that there is no connection at all – they just happen to work synchronistically because both are expressions of some underlying reality. Intermediate concepts make use of unknown physical principles, quantum mechanics in a whole range of guises and thermodynamics. In order to minimise confusion here, only a few specific theories will be mentioned; the general approaches will be subsumed under (a) 'traditional' dualism (briefly), (b) mainstream ideas about mind being an emergent property of brain function as it is presently conceived, (c) ideas which incorporate quantum mechanics. It will soon become apparent that there is overlap between all these categories, so they should be considered an aid to thought rather than rigorous or mutually exclusive.

TRADITIONAL DUALISM

This is the belief that awareness is an attribute of the immaterial soul possessed by each of us; the brain does not create awareness, but simply guides and is guided through links with the soul which alone is the seat of consciousness. It's an idea of great beauty and power, often given visible expression. When looking at a Piero della Francesca painting one can 'see' the numinous shining through. Everyone who has been in love has viewed the soul in their lover's eyes. Every psychotherapist of any worth has 'felt' some entity within his patient that escapes categories of biological, psychological or social determinism. Why, then, is it so deeply unpopular among many of the most thoughtful people in our culture?

It does not fit terribly well at first sight with the Newtonian world view, though Newton himself seems to have had no trouble with it (but perhaps his rather obsessive biblical studies indicate a hidden uneasiness). There's no obvious place for soul in his clockwork universe. C.S. Lewis (1953) pointed out that it was this very incompatibility which led Descartes to divorce the soul entirely from the body and allow the two to be linked only at the pineal gland. Previously soul, in one guise or another, had been assumed to be immanent throughout a universe which included our bodies and brains. Descartes went too far and, one suspects, so caused the downfall of the idea of soul. To be fair to him his actual views were more complex than those popularly attributed to him (Brown, 1985) but this complexity has usually been ignored and has thus failed to sustain his basic notion. Then, too, the wars of religion, the terrible simplicities of the naïvely religious, turned many more generous and ample minds against a whole set of ideas among which that of soul was included willy nilly.

Evidence was found to support Descartes' idea about the pineal quite soon after its publication. King (1686) dissected the brain of a man of whom, before death, it was said: 'his rational faculties seemed to be quite lost'. His pineal gland turned out to be 'petrified', the implication being that the link between the man's brain and soul must have been impaired before death. One can imagine that earnest Roentgenologists (radiologists) at the end of the nineteenth century might have added to the evidence using statistical arguments (they appear not to have done so because it was by then thought that such 'petrifaction' was normal); the pineal does in fact tend to calcify with age, this shows up on X-rays and should have obvious correlations with the loss of the soul's ability to influence the brain shown by the aged, with their decreased intellectual vigour, increased querulousness, etc.

Absurdities like this may well also have been responsible for a revulsion against the whole idea of soul, though not all share it. As mentioned in Chapter 2, Eccles (1989), a Nobel prizewinning neuroscientist, holds to something very like Descartes' conception which he shared with the famous Karl Popper. The main problem lies, not in the idea of soul as such, but in conceiving the nature of the links that it might have with the brain. Some ghostly capacity to influence probabilities, even if linked to ideas about quantum mechanics, does not entirely convince when approached from the top down (soul being a largely independent entity influencing the brain) as Eccles does. Bottom up approaches are less unsympathetic, particularly as there is such overwhelming evidence that the mind is in some sense a product of the brain. Who, then, needs souls? Only lovers and poets and it's mostly safe to ignore them – or so a thoroughgoing rationalist might claim.

THE MAINSTREAM

As streams do, this has meandered a good deal over the years and is now a lot more interesting than it was. Academic ideas about awareness tended to be simplistic in the days when behaviourism ruled, since to think about it at all was not respectable. As late as 1992, Searle thought it worth calling his book on consciousness *The **Rediscovery** of the Mind* (my bold italics). So impressed were many by computer technology that it was assumed that information processing was all, and that awareness was simply an epiphenomenon of the more elaborate sorts of processing. An example of the most basic unit of cognition, it was said, might be provided by a room thermostat which 'knows' if the room is too hot or too cold.

The Turing test provided additional justification for not thinking too deeply about awareness. Alan Turing in England (and Alonzo Church in America) were responsible for the mathematical theory which allowed the development of digital computers, all of which are examples of universal computing machines often referred to as Turing machines. The story of how he made a (perhaps the) major contribution to breaking enemy cyphers during the Second World War, and was subsequently hounded to suicide for his homosexuality, is now well known. The eponymous test arose from one of his speculations. He thought that digital computers would soon develop so far that people might not be able to distinguish between answers provided by the computer and those provided by a fellow human. Suppose one were to talk to some entity over the phone and, after detailed questioning, to decide that it was human, only to be told that: 'no, sorry, that was our computer'. If the two cannot be distinguished, what right has one to say that the computer is not just as conscious as the questioner? And, in that case, what's the point of thinking too much about awareness since it is either an epiphenomenon of computation whether by computers or by brains, or else it is not distinguishable from such computation and is, therefore, pointless? Incidentally, no computer has yet passed the Turing test but there seems no reason why it should not happen one day soon if anyone bothers to put enough effort into writing the appropriate programme and providing the computer with enough background information on which to draw. It's unlikely that anyone will bother as the Turing test, after dominating much of the thinking about consciousness for a decade or more up to the early 1980s, is now widely perceived as irrelevant.

The more interesting epoch in the history of ideas belonging to this paradigm arrived with something of a flourish occasioned by the publication in 1979 of Hofstadter's marvellous book (*Godel, Escher, Bach: An Eternal Golden Braid*). Witty, erudite and enthralling, it is best read in full. One cannot really do justice to it at second hand. What he does is to take Godel's mathematical proofs, especially his incompleteness theorem, Escher's lithographs of impossible scenes and objects and J.S. Bach's music to show how all three depend for their effectiveness on constant self-reference, self-reiteration and reflexive development. He then goes on to argue that consciousness is a product of similar self-referring organisational principles within the brain.

His *tour de force* is the section entitled 'Ant fugue', narrated in part by Aunt Hilary who turns out to be an anteater. He imagines his ant colony to be conscious, but its consciousness is based on patterns of activity in groups of ants not the activities of single ants (for ants read neurones). Aunt Hilary is benign, keeping the consciousness of the colony in trim by weeding out individual rogue ants that might threaten the evolution of the most desirable patterns. In fact the colony that she describes was a genius among ant colonies: then came a rainstorm one day which washed through the nest completely disrupting the activities within it. When they reformed, though the individual ants were the same, the patterns were different and the personality of the colony had totally changed!

It's a beguiling picture, and one which has had a good deal of influence. The most convincing development of it was made by Edelman (1989) who argued that consciousness emerges from patterns of 're-entrant' nervous activity between groups of neurones. 'The notion of re-entry extends well beyond those of simple feedback, feedforward, or recurrent circuits, and should not be confused with them' (Tononi *et al.*, 1992). The concept is in fact of detailed alignment of patterns of activity, constantly updated, between neuronal groups that may be quite remote from one another. A theory running along similar general lines to Edelman's, but couched in mainly psychological terms instead of mainly neurological ones, is due to Humphrey (1992). This book is memorable particularly for the many apt and beautiful quotations from English literature with which Humphrey embellishes his account.

This set of ideas is intriguing, ingenious and alluring but curiously insubstantial: one can never quite get a feeling of how awareness might actually emerge from all this reflexive activity. The Escher lithographs provide a most apt metaphor. The scenes or objects that they depict are fascinating, beautiful even, but they are illusions. They don't exist in three dimensions and never could.

Dennett (1991) is a philosopher who is a strong supporter of the Edelman-type line. He has many interesting and true things to say about the organisation of the neural functions which underpin mental life, but whenever he gets on to consciousness itself rhetoric and verbosity creep in. His argument can be (perhaps unfairly) simplified to:

clearly consciousness does arise from the sorts of neural behaviour that I've described, but these do not have any unique qualities that might differentiate mental life from brain activity, so you are mistaken when you think that your phenomenal experience is in any way special or as you conceive it to be, even though one has to agree that you do experience it as special.

Probably all discussions of awareness that use only this particular set of ideas must inevitably reach this dead end.

Meanwhile, the computer scientists have been going on from strength to strength, stimulated by the discovery that artificial intelligence is not easily achieved. You can get a digital computer to play grandmaster standard chess all right, but getting it to recognise a face is another matter. So they started to look at how the brain does things. Clearly, the brain does not have a central processor through which everything must go in sequence; instead there are many input and output channels that work in parallel. Moreover, the actual computational work in the brain appears to be achieved in messy networks where everything is connected to everything else. Already computers have been built which use parallel distributed processing to deal with inputs, though they do not have so many channels (yet) as does the brain. 'Neural networks' are also a hot topic, though few have been built; what has generally been done is to write programs for fast, sequential computers which allow them to behave as if they were small networks. Nevertheless, the behaviour of these simulations is interesting. They can learn from experience, for instance, without any guidance or a controlling program, and they can retain information about patterns of past activity in them for a considerable time until it gets overlaid. They are surprisingly brain-like in some important respects.

Extending this approach to cover awareness raises the question of why awareness should contain so little information when there is so much going on in the brain, but there is an answer to this well expressed by Baars (1993):

> Much of the nervous system can be viewed as a massively parallel, distributed system of highly specialized but unconscious processors. Conscious experience on the other hand is traditionally viewed as a serial *stream* that integrates different sources of information but is limited to only one internally consistent content at any given moment. Global Workspace theory suggests that conscious experience emerges from a nervous system in which multiple input processors compete for access to a broadcasting capability: the winning processor can disseminate its information *globally* throughout the brain. Global Workspace architectures have been widely employed in computer systems to integrate separate modules when they must work together to solve a novel problem or to control a coherent new response. The theory articulates a series of increasingly complex models, able to account for more and more evidence about conscious functioning, from perceptual consciousness to conscious problem-solving, voluntary control of action, and directed attention. Global Workspace theory is consistent with, but not reducible to, other theories of limited-capacity mechanisms. Global Workspace architectures must show competition for input to a neural global workspace and global distribution of its output. Brain structures that are demonstrably required for normal conscious experience can carry out these two functions.

All this provides too neat an explanation of our butterfly awareness's behaviour to be entirely wrong. Competing spatio-temporal functional units, queuing to occupy the workspace, could originate anywhere in the brain's patchwork quilt. Perhaps they always have to wait for up to half a second in the queue before entry.

Surely Baars must be correct, at least in general approach, about how the brain works but what about the mind? He has given extremely valuable insights into the underpinnings of mind but is only assuming that these underpinnings are enough to wholly account for conscious experience. Searle's (1990) 'Chinese room' argument has shown to the satisfaction of many people (as pointed out later, in Chapter 6, it's surprising that so many should be so satisfied with Searle's argument) that information processing, about which Baars is talking, and understanding occupy different realms. Maybe the Global Workspace is a sufficiently different realm but, if so, why is it? Then, of course, perceptual qualities do not appear to get a look-in in this sort of scheme. The information dealt with in consciousness no doubt gets there in the way that Baars suggests or something very like it, but the 'guts' of awareness, the sensuous immediacy of mental life, seems to demand something more. In essence, Baars is claiming that awareness is an epiphenomenon of a particular type of information processing (i.e. that occurring in a global workspace).

Arguments about whether consciousness is only epiphenomenal have gone on at tedious length for many years with the camps for and against about evenly balanced. Elitzur (1989) believed that he had shown that it must be efficacious if only because 'consciousness must be the reason why people are bothered by problems of consciousness' (a rather Hofstadter-like, reflexive proposal!), but this argument does not seem to have impressed those temperamentally in favour of epiphenomenalism, while those against it need no convincing. The airy abstractions of information processing theory appear to many not enough on their own to instantiate all the vivid earthiness of consciousness. Edelman claims that his approach is different from and more substantial than an information processing one, but when analysed it clearly belongs to the information processing continuum.

The future of the mainstream is of course uncertain, but one particularly intriguing channel may be leading it directly towards our next category of ideas. This is the concept of quantum computing, which has a lot of attractions for computer theorists who could in principle use the potentialities in the pre-collapse wave function to work out all possible answers to a problem at the same time. In effect, one would have a massively parallel machine without the need physically to build parallel channels. A quantum computer could therefore perform certain probabilistic tasks faster than any classical machine (Deutsch, 1985). It could also store and use information more efficiently than a classical machine (Ekert, 1994). None have yet been built, but the basic logic circuits for them have been designed and already machines are in use for absolutely secure encryption that depend on quantum principles; even an Alan Turing could not crack their cypher.

PENROSE

An Oxford mathematician whose interests range from the theory of black holes, on which he worked with Stephen Hawking, to making shapes that can completely cover a flat surface while forming patterns that never repeat themselves (he was able to reduce the number of different shapes needed to achieve this to only two; when the problem was first tackled, the number needed was 20,426, soon cut down to 104 then 6). He has also become much involved with the problems of mentality; an interest which seems to run in his family as his father made seminal contributions to studies of the genetics of mental disorder, particularly mental handicap.

One of the main themes of his book (*The Emperor's New Mind*, 1989) centres around how mathematicians can arrive as they do at truths. He argues that they cannot always do it by processes of logic or computation as currently understood. Logic is ruled out by Godel's incompleteness theorem which shows beyond doubt that any mathematical system complex enough to say anything of interest can be used to express truths that could never be proved from the axioms of the system. Computation is ruled out because it cannot deal with so-called non-recursive functions needed to arrive at some mathematical truths. All computation depends on the use of algorithms in Turing machines, but some essential computations can't be carried out because the necessary algorithms can't exist; for instance, it is inherently impossible to construct an algorithm which will allow one to discover whether a Turing machine computation will ever stop!

Therefore, says Penrose, the brains of mathematicians, and presumably other people too, can't be Turing machines. Maybe they are quantum computers instead. It's an intriguing possibility, though he has not proved it. The proof of Godel's theorem depends on expressing the rules of any mathematical system in the symbolism of the system and one could, so to speak, jack the whole symbolic level up by adding meta-rules in the same symbolism. The theorem still holds, but the level of abstraction can quickly become so great that mere humans, even mathematicians, could not necessarily discern any particular instances of limitations in one another's reasoning caused by it. We could be subject to Godel limitations without knowing it if our 'brain programming' is several steps up the meta-rule ladder. Another possible objection, hinted at by Penrose himself in his latest (1994) book, is that mathematicians may proceed by making *mistakes* which will inevitably include a few inadvertent truths whose validity can later be established by some sort of pseudo-Darwinian selection process. Ideal Turing machines don't make mistakes, so cannot progress towards truth in this way. Then, too, it seems to be in any case unlikely that quantum computers could solve non-recursive functions any better than classical ones (Deutsch, 1985), though they might well arrive at approximate answers faster – which could still be a considerable gain from an evolutionary point of view to any animal using quantum computing, provided the approximate answer was near enough correct to allow correct action.

Leaving these objections aside, a quantum computer calculation needs some sort of stopping criterion or the wave function would just go on evolving endlessly, multiplying possible answers. Collapse of the wave function provides an obvious read-out mechanism for such calculation. Of course, the major part of the calculation might have been carried out long before collapse by reduction of the probability amplitudes of incorrect answers to very low levels; collapse might only provide a sort of final 'endorsement' of the outcome of calculation (though there would always be some possibility of a less likely answer materialising instead of the main favourite). Penrose's suggestion is that collapse of this sort manifests itself in conscious decision-making. It will occur, according to his original collapse theory, when enough of the brain is involved in the calculation to allow differences between the possibilities in the relevant wave function to exceed the one graviton threshold (see Chapter 3). He estimated that quite a lot of brain would need to be involved before collapse is likely to happen since the relevant differences within the wave function depend mainly on different ion shifts across nerve cell membranes, and it would require a lot of ion shifts to amount to one graviton's worth. His new theory does not need such large energy differences to make collapse happen at a reasonable rate, say within a tenth of a second, but he still thinks that quite extensive brain areas might need to be involved in a pre-collapse superposition before read-out could be expected to happen.

It's not really necessary to propose any new physics, such as Penrose's gravitational collapse theory, in order to reach the view that conscious decision-making is likely to be the outcome of quantum field collapse. A respected Californian physicist (Stapp, 1994) has argued on a basis of traditional quantum theory only that particular conscious experiences, which of course include conscious decisions, should be considered outcomes of brain quantum events.

One can see that the Penrose/Stapp idea has possible links with the global workspace notion since both require competition among alternative possibilities, followed by a sort of 'crystallisation' when sufficiently extensive brain areas have become involved. The particular advantage of Penrose's approach, as we shall see in the next chapter, is that it gives a rationale for practical experimentation. Meanwhile, we are still left without any clear, concrete proposals about how consciousness might be instantiated.

QUANTUM CONSCIOUSNESS?

Even if thinking about consciousness *per se* does not necessarily make for unhappiness, you will almost certainly find that the application to it of some ideas about quantum mechanics will cause discomfort. The trouble is that one man's source of intellectual pain is another's marvellous provider of insight and enlightenment. Which particular ideas you find uncongenial probably depends more on your temperament than on the inherent worth of the ideas themselves – assuming, that is, that an idea has any worth independently of the mind that holds it. One could try to talk about more widely accepted and less widely accepted views, but nobody has done the surveys of opinion necessary to support this approach. It's probably best to describe the range that exists and pick out one's personal favourites while realising that they won't be everyone's cup of tea.

Early attempts to involve quantum theory in nervous activity tended to be made by people who disliked the idea of neural determinism and wanted to keep some place for 'free will'. They tended to concentrate on Heisenberg's uncertainty principle, especially the fact that the wave function of an electron occupies a considerable volume, so its position is uncertain, so it can theoretically appear in some unexpected part of a neurone which might, in certain critical circumstances, cause the neurone to fire so perhaps causing some unpredictable mental event. It was really all a bit laboured and painful from many people's point of view. Interestingly enough much of the steam has gone out of this approach since people have come to realise that neural activity is often chaotic and is therefore unpredictable for that reason: this despite the fact that the delicately balanced nature of chaotic systems actually makes it far more plausible that positional uncertainties could have the effect envisaged! As mentioned earlier, Eccles takes the not dissimilar view that mind influences brain by altering the probability of release of synaptic vesicles, which of course depends on electrical phenomena.

If the above can be regarded as a 'narrow' view of how quantum phenomena might be involved in mental function, there are also views that might be thought excessively broad, based on the philosophies of idealism and some aspects of Platonism. To them, consciousness is the primary reality, while matter is some sort of secondary manifestation of it. Although consciousness is basically universal, our individual minds appear to lead separate existences because of their involvement with matter. Quantum theory may be crucial to understanding exactly how consciousness relates to matter. Goswami (1990) is a recent, and unusually lucid, exponent of these views which certainly appeal to some temperaments and are of scientific value, too, as they are in principle refutable (see Chapter 5).

A more limited role is given to consciousness by Lockwood (1989) and Squires (1990). It is no longer the fount and origin of the material world, but is an operator nesting in the branches of everything that is possible and determining which branch shall be real for it. This idea has its origins in the long prevalent opinion that conscious observation is what collapses the wave function. When explored in detail it seems to lead fairly inevitably to a 'many worlds' view in some variant or other; Lockwood seems inclined to believe that one need not accept that all possible worlds share the same degree of physical reality, though a 'many biographies' view must be accepted – i.e. that one in fact lives all possible streams of experience though distinguishable streams are mutually inaccessible to one another. How this squares with a lack of physical separability between different worlds is not stated clearly. Although these are quite elegant intellectual structures (if one ignores the grotesque nature of their many worlds outcome), they are probably sterile as their validity is inherently untestable.

It's probably fair to say that all the ideas described hitherto in this Chapter about connections between awareness and quantum theory lack a quality that might be described as 'body', weight or perhaps commonsense plausibility. This applies particularly to Penrose (1989) who did not commit himself to any particular role for awareness but simply implied that conscious decision-making is in some way specially associated with wave function collapse. His latest views (see *Shadows of the Mind*, 1994) are more concrete and endorse Hameroff's notion, mentioned in Chapter 1 under 'exotica', that shape changes in tubulin molecules have computational functions and that quantum effects related to these may underpin consciousness. The next step is to look at ideas of this sort in more detail.

MARSHALL

Ian Marshall's ideas about consciousness, long in gestation, were first published in 1989, which seems to have been something of an *annus mirabilis* for the production of important works on this topic in England. It's tempting to think that this was the result of a natural intellectual reaction to the short-termism and mindless materialism of the Thatcher years. The ideas have been further developed in collaboration with Danah Zohar, his wife, who has described them and some of their implications in a couple of books for the general reader (Zohar, 1990 and Zohar and Marshall, 1993). It's the basic notions that we shall look at here: the implications will be discussed in a later chapter.

He argues that the unity combined with the complexity of conscious states is such as to be unexplainable in terms of any classical physical system. Of quantum systems, Bose–Einstein condensates have exactly the right characteristics to account for these properties. As was first proposed by Frohlich (1986), it is likely that such condensates occur between phonons generated by dipole oscillators in nerve cell (and other cell) membranes. These oscillators are electrically polarised molecules, proteins or glycoproteins, which span the cell membrane and will be affected by the trans-membrane voltage, and any changes in it. Therefore, consciousness could be, said Marshall, a manifestation of Bose–Einstein condensation instantiated, at least in humans, in this particular physical system.

The dipole oscillations occur at microwave frequencies, so, if the theory is right, consciousness and cellular processes generally might be expected to be particularly sensitive to applied microwaves of the same frequency. Though there's no evidence about consciousness itself, various cellular systems are greatly affected by narrow microwave frequency bands (Frohlich, 1986) while remaining unaffected by similar energies in neighbouring bands; nervous tissue, too, shows narrow frequency band effects (Adey, 1981). It therefore seems very probable that Frohlich systems, or something closely related to them, do actually occur in living organisms.

Marshall envisages the brain as being a bit like a hologram (which is the pattern of interference fringes recorded on a photographic plate when an object is illuminated by laser light). A 3D image of the object appears when the plate is lit by light of the same frequency as was used for recording and, interestingly, the whole image can be regained from any part of the plate, though the resolution is poorer the smaller the fragment of plate that is lit. Laser light is a Bose–Einstein condensate, so the idea is that the brain condensate, which comprises awareness, 'lights up' so to speak patterns of nervous activity to produce particular mental images or states. There is obviously room here for subtleties concerning whether the condensate might relate to current patterns of activity or records of past activity or both, but these are not pursued.

If one accepts the basic premise that consciousness is a manifestation of Bose–Einstein condensation in the brain, there is, nevertheless, room for doubt about some of the detail of Marshall's ideas. One such objection is primarily aesthetic; i.e that the Frohlich system seems inherently too messy to suffice. Vibrating dipoles in cell membranes must come in a variety of shapes and sizes, and one might anticipate that different sorts would condense in different circumstances, so perhaps undermining arguments for their importance from the unity of awareness. C.J.S. Clarke (unpublished paper, 1994) found mathematical evidence that the energy spectrum would be too widespread to allow condensation to occur in the way envisaged by Frohlich when he removed some of the simplifying assumptions that Frohlich had made in his own mathematical treatment.

This is not a fatal objection to the whole concept since, as was mentioned in Chapter 1, there is a much neater proposal due to Del Giudice *et al.* (1986). This is that hydrolysis of ATP or GTP molecules (the main cellular power source) generates solitons in long chains of protein molecules which in turn cause dipole vibration in so-called 'vicinal' polarised water adherent to the protein. This then generates phonons able to form Bose condensates in the manner envisaged by Frohlich. There seems to be no detailed mathematical treatment yet of the feasibility of this proposal but it certainly looks as if it should result in a narrow energy spectrum (because all solitons would be equally energetic). There is something deeply appealing about the notion that consciousness might ultimately be based on the behaviour of water; it has all sorts of poetic resonances. Even if its allure should prove false, however, there are the other candidates for undergoing condensation referred to in Chapter 1 (solitons themselves or Goldstone bosons).

Yet another candidate has been proposed very recently by Jibu and colleagues (1993); Hameroff was one of the co-authors. They suggested that the relevant Bose condensates might be of *photons*, the particles of light, instead of phonons which are particles of mechanical vibration. Their calculations indicate that the interior of microtubules, which are filled mainly with water, could generate coherent photons just like laser light. The process of generation would depend on a phenomenon called superradiance instead of the more familiar lasing, but the outcome would be the same. They create a beguiling picture in which microtubules act as sources and waveguides for light showing long-range coherence effects, thus implying that the brain is a giant, optical, quantum computer.

A greater problem for Marshall than uncertainty about the detail of how condensates might arise is his proposal that consciousness is based on a system involving extensive areas of the brain, or even the whole brain, and operating at microwave frequencies. It ought, therefore, to be capable of dealing with far larger amounts of information than the unconscious, 'classical' neurological systems which work at only a few hertz and are probably more subject to spatial constraints. However, there is overwhelming evidence that exactly the reverse is true; unconscious systems can deal with vastly more information than conscious ones. Jibu and colleages also use the hologram analogy, which is even more apt in relation to their proposal. The brain that they picture should, however, be able to handle absolutely incredible amounts of information consciously.

Since conscious, and even unconscious, rates of information processing are much less than ought to be the case in either of these theories, and especially in Jibu's version, the hologram picture has to be jettisoned except, perhaps, in relation to memory mechanisms. We need to think of awareness in new terms even though we can leave open the question of whether it may be based on phonons or photons, solitons or Goldstone bosons; at a fundamental level, and in their ability to create condensates, these particles are not so different from one another as is implied by the differences between their names.

It seems likely that the formation of any particular condensate in the brain is a slow process, though whether it could take as much as the 400 msecs or so implied by Libet's findings (Chapter 2) must remain open to doubt. Classical neuronal systems have to activate themselves, sufficient dipole vibrational energy, or whatever, must be generated and then a condensate can crystallise to link the relevant neurones. If Penrose's collapse theory (see Chapter 3) is correct then additional delays would be introduced since condensation would not occur until some relevant gravitational energy difference criterion had been exceeded, and this might depend mainly on alternative ion shifts across cell membranes (at least until gross blood flow changes had time to occur). All the same, it's not easy to see where a delay of as long as nearly half a second could come from. Penrose (1994) speculated that there might be something inherently 'fuzzy' about the relationship of consciousness to time which would necessitate taking figures like 'a 400 msec. delay' with a pinch of salt.

In spite of doubts like these, the view that we are having to adopt (*pace* Marshall) is that, if awareness has anything to do with Bose–Einstein condensation, it must be envisaged as being made up of a succession of extended objects in the brain which are likely to succeed one another at quite a slow rate. The objects will consist of spatially-structured patterns of activity, their actual shape dependent on the position of the particular neurones contributing energy to them. It must be remembered, however, that each object will be single and indivisible in an even stronger sense than a picture, say, or a vase is a single object; it is actually meaningless to talk about separate particles in a Bose–Einstein condensate.

BRAIN QUANTUM OBJECTS AND THE QUALIA PROBLEM

A main reason for pursuing ideas like Marshall's is the hope that they might lead to some sort of understanding of how experience can have the qualities that we all perceive. It's worth dwelling on a couple of rather unusual experiences to get a firmer picture of what needs to be explained. One is synaesthaesia in which the qualities of one sensory modality are experienced in terms of another modality. The wine buff's phrase – 'This is a well-rounded little claret' – is a relatively trivial example, but there are people who consistently experience particular colours when hearing particular sounds, for example, or get tactile sensations associated with tastes. The whole phenomenon has been described at length by Cytowic (1994). That this sort of thing happens suggests that what is going on in the brain determines the quality of an experience, not what is going on in the outside world or in the sensory organs.

My second example suggests the opposite – i.e. that the locus of awareness is not necessarily always in the brain. Tart (1993) discusses 'out of the body' experiences and quotes a description given by someone who was using a rather sophisticated remote control robot which gave tactile as well as visual feed-back:

I began to look through the eyes of the robot. The world looked like the world would look if I was located twelve feet to the left of my body, where the robot was located. . . . The strangest moment was when Dr Tachi told me to look to my right. There was a guy in a dark blue suit and light blue painted shoes reclining in a dentist's chair. He was looking to his right, so I could see the bald spot on the back of his head. He looked like me, and abstractly I understood that he was me, but I know who me is and me is *here*. He, on the other hand, was *there*.

Velmans (1992), who does not discuss quantum concepts, has a model of perception that seems to allow room for both the types of experience mentioned above:

> Provided that the conditions for conscious experience are met, visual processing results in a visual experience of that event *projected* (reflexively) to the judged location of the initiating cause. This is neither a 'ghostly' percept of the event in some non-extended mind, nor a neural representation. It is simply the event as-perceived. There is no experience of the event in the mind or brain *in addition to* the external event as-perceived. . . . The paper reviews evidence that similar projective processes operate (reflexively) in other sense modalities to produce what we normally think of as the external 'physical' world.

A problem with this model is that it is not clear how the 'event as-perceived' could be differentiated from brain processes of some sort. It is here that quantum concepts make the crucial difference. As Stapp (1985) points out, wave function collapse is inherently non-local. If it occurs in a brain, as well as entangling outside objects with which the brain is currently interacting, it will also involve (as shown by the experimental results that contravened Bell's inequality) particles with which certain relevant constituents of that brain have interacted in the past. This allows us to view Velmans's 'event as-perceived' as a composite object assembled from components both belonging to the brain and from the external world. It seems fair to conclude, at the simplest level, that when we experience redness, for example, it's not just a matter of some neurological symbol giving rise to the experience; rather, the experience is a representation of an inherent quality of that particular wavelength of light, relative to other wavelengths capable of interacting with the retina of the eye (though an unusual nervous system could be wired so as to represent it in a way that might produce an experience of a particular tone, say, instead of a colour). A memory of a colour is not in principle different from the 'present' experience of that colour, not only because of Libet's findings, but also because there is not necessarily any time limit on the ability of phenomena in the external world that once related to the brain to also connect with present wave function collapse in the brain.

There is a difficulty in applying Stapp's argument to the concept of awareness given here. This is to do with the fact that there are three different types of 'particle' to consider; the Bose condensates themselves as single quantum objects, the phonons (or whatever) which condense to form them and the particles of the molecules from which the phonons originate. It's not clear which of these should be regarded as having relevant non-local interactions with particles outside the brain. However, the (shortened for the sake of clarity) chain of photon arriving at eye, electron in optic nerve, phonon in visual cortex, Bose condensate involving visual cortex, is probably sufficient (so at least Penrose has implied) to establish a non-local link between photon and condensate. It looks as if there should be time constraints of some sort on the link, though, as two of the particles involved (condensates and phonons) are so ephemeral. Unfortunately, everything to do with time in quantum theory is unclear, so nothing definite can be said about this. While we're on this subject, it's worth noting that long relationship chains may sometimes be short-circuited; maybe, for instance, two peoples' Bose condensates truly become one on those rare occasions when all sense is lost of where 'I' end and 'you' begin. Most people have occasionally experienced this when making love, but it can also happen in other types of relationship. Those who watched the figure skaters Torvill and Dean at their best will remember that they often seemed to merge into one – maybe that's just what they really did.

It thus seems likely that there is quite a strong sense in which our experience is directly of aspects of the world as they really are or were. The usual assumption that all experience is only of indirect neural representations of the world may well be incorrect. This is not really a very new idea. St Thomas Aquinas (died 1274), following Aristotle, was probably saying something very similar when he hypothesised that human awareness is due to an internalisation of the 'forms' of external objects. The difference now is that quantum theory lends it plausibility after long centuries during which the Newtonian world view had rendered it inconceivable to any up-to-date thinker.

One can perhaps see how this view might begin to account for perceptual qualities, but what about other types of experience? A feeling of pity, say, or a conviction that God exists. Well, individual brains relate to each other as well as to the inanimate world, and their interrelationships will also be quantum integrated at various levels (dependent on the closeness of their previous interactions). When dealing with emotions and beliefs, we are in what Popper and Eccles (1977) describe as 'World 3' – that of human culture. Although in one sense immaterial, it is nevertheless instantiated in a whole range of physical systems, including other people's brains, which can in principle have similar, if more subtle, relationships to our own brains as red-coloured objects. Like many ideas arising from quantum theory, a seemingly fairly innocuous first step can quickly lead one into very deep waters indeed. We have already reached the concept of culture as some sort of quasi-object; Jungian-like ideas about racial subconsciousness may be only a further step away. This sense of being carried along further and faster than one might wish to go is thoroughly uncongenial to many temperaments, which may account for a reluctance that is often met to allow that quantum theory, the truest if the strangest description of nature that we have, must apply also to our brains.

To summarise, the claim is that awareness consists of a succession of quasi-objects materialising in the brain (at a rate, probably, of around ten per second). These will differ in shape according to which parts of the brain contribute to them and their topological structure will bear a direct relationship to whatever aspect of the world they are reflecting. Awareness is, in other words, a mirror which can reflect basic qualities like the colour and shape of an object but also more abstract things such as emotional tones. From the point of view of an outside observer, however, it could be difficult to tell where the 'real' object ends and the reflection begins, as when one sees mountains reflected in a lake on a windless day. The frame of the mirror can be thought of as the self or 'I', or perhaps 'I' sometimes takes the form of a systematic distortion of the reflecting surface.

CONCLUSIONS

We have in this book singled out various aspects of awareness for special attention, while emphasising the impediments to constructive thought introduced by uncertainty over the role of memory. The special areas are:

1　Its subjective 'feel'; the qualia problem.
2　Its spatial structure; the binding problem.
3　Libet's findings concerning its timing.
4　The slow rate at which it can deal with information.
5　Its energy requirements.
6　Its vulnerability to anaesthetics and to fragmentation.

How well do the various theories described in this chapter deal with these features of consciousness?

Cartesian dualism has to be regarded as a non-contender despite its long history and aesthetic appeal. By placing the soul in a realm of its own, it explains everything and nothing. A complete theory of the mind, when such is available, may conceivably entail acceptance of the idea of soul by a process of exclusion. But, in the meantime, to use the idea could only impede progress towards a more complete under-standing. Its heuristic value is analogous to that of Freudianism in psychiatry which may perhaps have stimulated some people's imagina-tions but, nevertheless, led them down all sorts of conceptual and therapeutic blind alleys. Those enamoured of traditional dualism can always comfort themselves with the reflection that it may well in the end turn out to have expressed an aspect of the truth. However, we are concerned here with the utility of ideas and their relative truth, not their absolute truth.

The ideas which are testable and are therefore the main contenders can be characterised as those belonging to the Hofstadter/Edelman (HE) paradigm and those belonging to the Penrose/Marshall (PM) paradigm. It should be said at once that HE ideas have been enormously more useful than PM ones hitherto in that they have provided a framework for huge quantities of extremely productive research. But what about the understanding necessary for future productivity? Will the Prime Minister overtake His Excellency in power?

As far as the subjective 'feel' of experience is concerned, it is probably fair to say that all attempts to apply the HE paradigm in explanation have a 'thin' and unconvincing quality; one can see that they might have substance, but when one tries to grasp or get to grips with it there is nothing there. As the application of the PM paradigm to the same problem has just been described in the previous section, the reader can judge for him/herself whether it is any less insubstantial.

In relation to the spatial structure of awareness, PM theories have a clear advantage; they envisage the formation of unified objects in the brain which not only reflect features of the external world but in a rather deep sense *are* aspects of those features. HE theories must rely on stories to do with correlated EEG activity solving the binding problem which again lack substance. The correlated activity occurs but, in PM terms, is not sufficient on its own (it could be a result of, or more likely a pre-requisite for, extensive wave function collapse).

Libet's findings cause problems for PM theories though they are not insuperable. Extending HE ideas by using the 'global workspace' notion gives a more natural explanation. The workspace could be conceived as a *quantum* entity, but this multiplies entities in a way that should be avoided unless necessitated by experimental evidence.

The puzzles surrounding the fact that consciousness deals with information so slowly are probably related to the 'Libet' ones and are also more naturally treated by HE theories (despite Edelman's own dislike of the notion of information processing in relation to his ideas!).

The energy requirements of awareness can be explained equally well at present by both sets of ideas, though the PM explanation is a bit crisper and so may be preferred by some on aesthetic grounds.

The evidence from the action of anaesthetics is weak (see note) but, as Hameroff (1994) points out, favours PM theories because one would expect on HE theories that they would act at receptor sites or on ion channels which seems not to be the case. On PM theories they should act on other proteins or perhaps on vicinal water (which, surprisingly, is a *good* solvent for them – see Clegg, 1983). On the other hand, the fact that awareness can so readily be fragmented in hysteria, psychoses and brain damage would seem to fit more naturally and economically with HE ideas.

The distribution of intellectual honours between the two paradigms appears fairly even at present. Which is preferred on the evidence to date will depend partly on individual views about how well PM ideas account for the subjective aspects of awareness. Of course, temperament and previous training, nature and nurture, are likely to influence preference more strongly still. The experimental evidence that needs to be considered is set out in the next Chapter.

NOTE

There's no evidence that anaesthetics, in the doses used in clinical practice, affect classical, HE-type neurotransmission. They could well, however, interfere with van der Waals forces important to quantum or computational functions of microtubules (Penrose, 1994). The problem with this interpretation is that anaesthetics usually make people inert; they *don't*, except very rarely, turn patients into automata or robots as would be expected if their sole function is to abolish awareness while not affecting other brain activities. One could get round this by claiming that quantum-level happenings are essential for getting the brain to do anything other than perform its vegetative functions (e.g. respiration), but such a claim would be contrary to all the evidence outlined in Chapters 1 and 2 that many, or even most, brain functions are *unconscious*. In our present state of ignorance, the most likely theory about how anaesthetics might work still seems to be that they may interfere with some specific (but unknown) type of neurotransmission in the brain stem 'machines' which support cortical activity in general, including consciousness.

REFERENCES

Adey, W.R. (1981) 'Tissue Interactions with Non-ionizing Electromagnetic Fields', *Physiological Reviews* 61(2), 435–513.

Baars, B.J. (1993) 'How Does a Serial, Integrated and Very Limited Stream of Consciousness Emerge from a Nervous System that is Mostly Unconscious, Distributed, Parallel and of Enormous Capacity', in *Experimental and Theoretical Studies of Consciousness*, CIBA Symposium No. 174, Wiley: Chichester.

Brown, T.M. (1985) 'Descartes, Dualism and Psychosomatic Medicine', in *The Anatomy of Madness*, W.F. Bynum, R. Porter and M. Shepherd (eds), Tavistock Publications: London.

Burns, J.E. (1990) 'Contemporary Models of Consciousness', Part 1, *Journal of Mind and Behaviour* 11(2), 153–72.

Clarke, C.J.S. (1994) 'Coupled Molecular Oscillators Do Not Admit True Bose Condensations' (to appear in *Journal of Physics A.*)

Clegg, J.S. (1983) 'Intracellular Water, Metabolism and Cell Architecture', Part 2, in *Coherent Excitations in Biological Systems*, H. Frohlich and F. Kremer (eds), Springer-Verlag: Berlin.

Cytowic, R. (1994), *The Man Who Tasted Shapes*, Abacus Books: London.

Del Giudice, E., Doglia, S., Milani, M. and Vitiello, G. (1986) 'Collective Properties of Biological Systems: Solitons and Coherent Electric Waves in a Quantum Field Theoretical Approach', in *Modern Bioelectrochemistry*, F. Gutmann and H. Keyzer (eds), Plenum: New York.

Dennett, D.C. (1991) *Consciousness Explained*, Penguin Books: Harmondsworth.

Deutsch, D. (1985), 'Quantum Theory, the Church-Turing Principle and the Universal Quantum Computer', *Proceedings of Royal Society of London* 400, 97–117.

Eccles, J.C. (1989) *Evolution of the Brain: Creation of the Self*, Routledge: London.

Edelman, G.M. (1989) *The Remembered Present: A Biological Theory of Neural Darwinism*, Basic Books: New York.

Ekert, A. (1994) 'Shannon's Theorem Revisited', *Nature* 367, 513–14.

Elitzur, A.C. (1989) 'Consciousness and the Incompleteness of the Physical Explanation of Behaviour', *Journal of Mind and Behaviour* 10(1), 1–20.

Frohlich, H. (1968) 'Long-range Coherence and Energy Storage in Biological Systems', *International Journal of Quantum Chemistry* 11, 641–9.

Frohlich, H. (1986) 'Coherent Excitations in Active Biological Systems', in *Modern Bioelectrochemistry*, F. Gutmann and H. Keyzer (eds), Plenum: New York.

Goswami, A. (1990) 'Consciousness in Quantum Physics and the Mind-Body Problem', *Journal of Mind and Behaviour* 11(1), 75–96.

Hameroff, S.R. (1994) 'Quantum Coherence in Microtubules: A Neural Basis for Emergent Consciousness?', *Journal of Consciousness Studies* 1(1), 91–118.

Hofstadter, D.R. (1979) *Godel, Escher, Bach: An Eternal Golden Braid*, Penguin Books: Harmondsworth.

Honderich, T. (1987) 'Mind, Brain and Self-conscious Mind', in *Mindwaves*, C. Blakemore and S. Greenfield (eds), Basil Blackwell: Oxford.

Humphrey, N. (1992) *A History of the Mind*, Chatto & Windus: London.

Jibu, M., Hagan, S., Hameroff, S.R., Pribram, K.H. and Yasue, K. (1993) 'Quantum Optical Coherence in Cytoskeletal Microtubules: Implications for Brain Function', reprint to be published in *Biosystem*.

King, E. (1686) 'A Relation of a Petrified Glandula Pinealis, Lately Found in the Dissection of a Brain', *Philosophical Transactions* 16, 228–31.

Lewis, C.S. (1953) *Poetry and Prose in the Sixteenth Century*, Clarendon Press: Oxford.

Lockwood, M. (1989) *Mind, Brain and the Quantum: the Compound I*, Basil Blackwell: Oxford.

Marshall, I.N. (1989) 'Consciousness and Bose-Einstein Condensates', *New Ideas in Psychology* 7(1), 73–83.

Penrose, R. (1989) *The Emperor's New Mind*, Oxford University Press.

Penrose, R. (1994) *Shadows of the Mind*, Oxford University Press.

Popper, K.R. and Eccles, J.C. (1977) *The Self and its Brain*, Springer International: New York.

St Thomas Aquinas (1991 edn) *Summa Theologiae. A Concise Translation*, T. McDermott (ed.), Methuen: London.

Searle, J.R. (1990), 'Who is Computing with the Brain?', *Behavioural and Brain Sciences* 13(4), 632–41.

Searle, J.R. (1992) *The Rediscovery of the Mind*, MIT Press: Cambridge, Mass. and London.

Squires, E. (1990) *Conscious Mind in the Physical World*, Adam Hilger: Bristol.

Stapp, H.P. (1985) 'Consciousness and Values in the Quantum Universe', *Foundations of Physics* 15(1), 35–47.

Stapp, H.P. (1994) 'The Integration of Mind into Physics', Paper presented at a University of Maryland conference on Fundamental Problems in Quantum Theory, 18–22 June 1994.

Tart, C.T. (1993) 'Mind Embodied: Computer Generated Virtual Reality as a New, Dualistic-Interactive Model for Transpersonal Psychology', in *Cultivating Consciousness*, K.R. Rao (ed.), Praeger: Westport and London.

Tononi, G., Sporns R. and Edelman, G.M. (1992) 'The Problem of Neural Integration: Induced Rhythms and Short-Term Correlations', in *Induced Rhythms in the Brain*, E. Basar and T.H. Bullock (eds), Birkhauser: Boston.

Velmans, M. (1992) 'Synopsis of "Consciousness, Brain and the Physical World"', *Philosophical Psychology* 5, 155–82.

Zohar, D. (1990) *The Quantum Self*, Bloomsbury: London.

Zohar, D. and Marshall, I. (1993) *The Quantum Society*, Bloomsbury: London.

5 On the track of awareness

Clearly, there is still much uncertainty about the nature of our butterfly. Is it the fragile by-product of evanescent patterns of self-referential electrochemical activity in the brain only? Or, hatched from such a source, does it take on a life of its own spreading its wings across the universe? The contrast between these two views is large and ought to have observable consequences.

One such consequence may be the very existence of science itself. In philosophical mood, scientists have often commented on the strangeness of the fact that symbolic processes in their own heads can so often reflect recherché truths about the nature of the real world. Indeed, some have gone so far as to take the rather solipsistic view that there is no fixed reality and no hard and fast laws of nature: science simply creates its own reality as it goes along. Although this view may have a limited validity, it's hard to believe that it is wholly correct. On the other hand, there is no puzzle if the quantum view of consciousness (the PM paradigm) is correct since, on it, the mental symbols and the natural phenomena to which they refer will in quite a strong sense *be the same*, provided the symbols are derived from accurate observation and are not too distorted by cultural influences. It's true that the direction of any scientist's gaze, and his particular focus on things, *is* always strongly influenced by cultural factors but that's a separate issue. Since the scientist, if he is a good one, directly partakes of the nature of what he studies, there is no great surprise when he arrives at the truth about it.

Of course, arguments like this, though sometimes valid, rarely carry much conviction and are particularly unlikely to do so in our present context since we are talking about awareness studying awareness whose nature it already shares. This involves Hofstadter-type reflection with a vengeance, and one could trust no line of thought that followed it for more than a step or two. What's needed are simple, objective tests to differentiate between the two paradigms.

A possible approach is to take a single aware system and pare it down as much as possible to ascertain the precise site (in anatomical or functional terms) of its awareness. This method is the one advocated by Crick and Koch (1992). They start off with a rousing peroration from which I cannot resist quoting excerpts here: 'The overwhelming question in neurobiology today is the relation between the mind and the brain' and '. . . until recently most cognitive scientists ignored consciousness, as did almost all neuroscientists. The problem was felt to be either purely "philosophical" or too elusive to study experimentally . . . In our opinion such timidity is ridiculous . . .'. They go on to suggest further study of the visual system from this point of view because a great deal is already known about it and some of the right experimental techniques are already in place. They believe that there is some preliminary evidence to indicate that visual awareness may be especially associated with the pyramidal cells in layer 5 of the visual cortex. Approaches like this are likely to be fruitful, but may take a long while to bear fruit. In a sense they are the safe option.

There is a more direct route to the goal of distiguishing between our two main paradigms: namely, to ascertain whether brains ever behave in the sort of way that might be expected of a quantum object and, if so, whether this behaviour seems to be specially associated with awareness. The holism and non-locality characteristic of quantum systems have no precise classical equivalents and, if either were to be shown to occur in relation to activities involving awareness, the HE paradigm would be refuted.

When translated into practical experiments, holism implies that the entire set-up will influence whatever is to be measured and non-locality implies that spatial separation between parts of the set-up will not modify the constraints introduced by holism. It is important to remember that non-locality effects *cannot* be used to actively transmit information instantaneously from one part of a system to another, which would contravene both special and general relativity. However, changes in one part of a system will nevertheless be instantaneously correlated with those in another and there is nothing to stop an experimenter spotting the correlations, however far apart the system components may be, provided he does not expect to do so at more than light speed.

It has also been suggested that quantum superpositions in relation to awareness may be detectable either in perceptual systems (Woo, 1981) or in relation to slight modifications of Marcel-type experiments on words with more than one meaning (McCarthy and Goswami,

1991). However, it seems very unlikely indeed that the consequences of superposition could ever be unambiguously distinguished from those of classical parallel processing, except through the non-locality effects that have already been mentioned, since quantum computing in superpositions is simply a method of carrying out parallel processing using only one physical channel instead of multiple channels. There might well be interference effects in quantum computations, but the same could be expected in any system recording the outcome of classical parallel computations and it would probably be impossible in practice to distinguish the two different sorts of interference.

Such evidence as there is derives from three categories of experiment: (1) EEG coherence studies, (2) the 'Southampton' experiments, (3) some so-called 'psi' (parapsychology) experiments. The Southampton tests will be described at length, not because they are more important or convincing than the others, but because I can report from first-hand experience some of the excitements and frustrations associated with work in this field. Discussing 'psi' experiments at all will undermine any residual credibility that I may have in some circles. However, some good work has in fact been carried out in this field, interesting ideas have arisen from it and in any case it is worth taking to heart Crick and Koch's comment on the undesirability of being timid.

EEG COHERENCE STUDIES

As was mentioned in Chapter 2, EEG coherence studies are now an important method for looking at how different parts of a single brain interrelate. They have led to the conclusion that one has to think of brain activity in terms of spatio-temporal functional units. However, exactly the same methods can be used to examine the degree of coherence between activity in two (or more) different brains and this is what Orme-Johnson *et al.* (1982) did.

Their reason for doing so was somewhat 'Californian' (though in fact they were based in Iowa). They were interested in transcendental meditation (TM), and especially in an apparently valid observation that local crime rates tended to decrease in an area in which enough people were carrying out TM. Sceptical readers will be glad to learn that this was NOT because you cannot commit a crime while actually engaged in TM; the meditators and the criminals were in fact different people. Anyhow, they decided to see whether the practice of TM has any observable remote effect on the EEG and used inter-subject coherence as a measure.

Subjects were placed in separate rooms with no intercommunication possible and were asked to meditate. Coherence measures between the subjects were obtained; the comparisons were between coherence at ordinary times and at times when 2500 meditators were having a mass meditate in a town 1170 miles away. Inter-subject coherence was significantly greater, especially at around alpha frequencies, at times when the 2500 were actually undertaking TM.

The obvious question to ask here is whether the subjects knew about the 2500 and about when they would be doing their stuff. Although quite elaborate randomised timing procedures were used to start the subjects' own TM sessions, this question was not addressed in the paper so one must remain very sceptical about its authors' conclusion that they had demonstrated the existence of some sort of non-local consciousness field.

A later, rather small, study from the same centre (Travis and Orme-Johnson, 1989) appeared to show that changes in the coherence of a meditator's EEG may cause changes in non-meditator's coherence, even when there is no possibility of any physical communication between the two, the effect being maximal for meditator's coherence changes in the 5.7 to 8.5 hz frequency band (analyses were made for 0.94 hz intervals). Most of the possible flaws in methodology seem to have been recognised and addressed in this study.

Working in a different centre, Grinberg-Zylberbaum and Ramos (1987) showed that subjects' inter-hemispheric correlation measures tended to converge when they felt that they were in communication with one another, even though there was apparently no electrical, acoustical or other obvious means by which they could communicate.

None of these studies are particularly convincing on their own or even as a group. They would need to be replicated in a number of different centres, and made acceptable to the referees of journals other than the one in which all three were published, before one could give them much credence. However, the methodology is interesting and, if the results did prove replicable, could be further developed. The Iowa group are inclined to attribute their findings to the existence of a universal field of consciousness of the type envisaged by Goswami (see Chapter 4). The others propose a 'neuronal field' based on unknown physical principles. However, it seems quite likely that 'ordinary' quantum non-locality considerations could account for the findings if they are in fact valid. As non-locality would only be influential between subjects who had had previous associations of some sort, it ought to be possible to devise experiments to see whether it does provide the best explanation of any positive findings.

THE SOUTHAMPTON EXPERIMENTS

The publication of Penrose's *The Emperor's New Mind* (1989) seven years ago gave a great fillip to people vaguely dissatisfied with the ideas about consciousness which were then prevalent in scientific and medical circles. They amounted to a rather inchoate version of the HE paradigm (see Chapter 4, conclusions). Not only did this book offer much broader and more satisfying (to some) horizons, but the ideas in it looked as if they might actually be *testable*.

Our problem in Southampton, then, was to test them without benefit of a research grant or much time, since we all had busy full-time jobs. One approach that was considered and abandoned was to induce presumed superpositions in people's visual areas by getting them to look at ambiguous pictures – the drawings that can be seen either as a man's face or as a seated girl, either as a duck or a rabbit, etc. – and then ascertain whether non-locality effects between subjects could be observed resulting in a particular perception. The idea was quickly abandoned both because the necessary statistics and control experiments would be horrific and because the whole thing smacked so much of a telepathy experiment (not a respectable line of enquiry!). Perhaps, on the other hand, something could be done with microwaves to interfere with Marshall's Bose–Einstein condensates; a possibility quickly rejected as certainly technically difficult and probably unethical.

In the end, we settled on something of an outside chance (Nunn *et al.*, 1994) because it was technically feasible and promised unambiguous results (we were naïve in those days). It will be remembered that measurement of an observable is what is thought to collapse the wave function, though what 'measurement' means is open to a very wide range of interpretations. Taking an EEG can be regarded as measuring some hypothetical brain quantum fields, i.e. those which result in different brain electrical states according to which possibility in a field becomes manifest. Suppose that a quantum field contains two possibilities: (1) I'm going to move my hand, (2) I'm not going to move my hand. An EEG recording from the relevant piece of motor cortex will vary according to which outcome actually occurs, and so can be regarded as performing a quantum measurement.

It's doubtful whether one could construct a valid test based on this fact in relation to most theories about precisely what collapses the wave function because one would have to think about neighbouring bits of brain also 'measuring' collapse in the motor cortex, which not only leads to an infinite regress (that indicator of conceptual error), but also would be likely to swamp any effect due to the EEG. Penrose's own theory (and just possibly some others) is different in that his gravitational criterion for collapse has the consequence that EEG pen movement would be significant because it would literally outweigh collapse induced by local changes in the brain. There's no classical theory on which taking an EEG should have the least direct effect on brain function. We therefore thought that, if we could observe such an effect, we would show that quantum principles are important to aspects of brain function and, if we did not find an effect, we would go quite a way towards refuting Penrose's theory. Frankly, we expected to refute Penrose.

Next was the problem of what sort of effect of collapse of hypothetical fields on brain function to look for, given that no one knows what consciousness actually does or even if it is efficacious at all. Penrose's theory in its original version suggested that collapse will occur sooner when an EEG is being taken from a relevant brain area, so reaction times seemed a sensible thing to look at. However, in view of Libet's work, it seemed safer to throw in other measures too since his findings indicate that there is no simple relationship between action and awareness. It was just as well that we did so because the latest version of Penrose's theory no longer predicts a specific effect on reaction times. Moreover, awareness might either inhibit or facilitate a response and there was no guarantee that different subjects would use the same strategy in this respect.

Eventually, we cobbled together a test using old bits of apparatus that we were able to borrow. The age of the EEG machine (about twenty years) was actually an advantage as its pen recorders were a good deal heavier than the ink jets used by modern machines. Subjects were to respond with their right thumbs to some out of a series of random digits flashed on to a small screen. Doing this is mainly a left hemisphere task. Meanwhile, they were given a distraction in the form of music played to their left ears (people who are not trained musicians tend to use their right hemispheres to deal with music, and about 90 per cent of input to the left ear goes to the right hemisphere). All were right-handed as left-handers sometimes use unexpected brain areas for doing things. Outcome measures were averaged reaction times, proportion of target numbers missed and proportion of incorrect hits on non-targets. Meanwhile, the EEG was recorded in random sequence from the right side of the brain or from the left side (with a control condition of no EEG recording). The whole set-up was just about good enough to make the expected negative result meaningful. It was not good enough to make any positive result a firm indication of the occurrence of quantum effects rather than some type of experimental error.

It was quite a boring test for both subjects and experimenter. Nevertheless, 28 staff members from the Southampton psychiatric services nobly undertook it. The minds of two were obviously elsewhere as they made more than 30 per cent errors, so their results were not used; the remainder tried hard. The first five to be tested missed significantly more target numbers when their EEGs were being recorded from the right. Because we had been thinking in terms of global electrical states of each hemisphere as the relevant 'measurable', the left-side EEG was recorded between occipital and frontal electrodes (the right was always between posterior temporal and parietal electrodes). As a result, there was more machine noise during left-sided recordings (because the machine was picking up frontalis muscle activity), and perhaps this was causing the surprise result. So the left electrode placements were altered to match those on the right in the next five tests (each subject was tested only once). This group showed very significantly *fewer* misses during left-sided recording. There was no obvious way of explaining this in terms of experimental error, so it was all quite exciting. If we had realised that activity in the relevant bits of the brain 'patchwork quilt' was the electrical variable of importance, rather than global hemispheric states, we would have predicted that moving the electrodes should alter the results obtained; as it was, we did not realise this until it was forced on us. Further batches of tests confirmed our findings. It was disappointing that we had discovered no differences in reaction times, but clearly what had been found merited more careful investigation.

There were various things to be done; testing had to be fully automated so that the experimenter had no way of influencing performance; the EEG machine had to be put in a different room from the testee; control tests were needed to ascertain whether electrical or acoustic feedback from the apparatus could be influencing results. We settled on two tests: (a) having to respond with the right hand to certain words out of a small vocabulary flashed in random order on to a computer screen, while listening to music delivered to the left ear. We hoped that this would use just about the same brain areas as were involved in our original number test, and (b) responding with the left hand to certain pairs of patterns out of a small library of pairs of four by four chequerboard patterns, while listening to a recorded lecture delivered to the right ear. This was intended to be a sort of mirror image of the first test as far as relevant brain areas for doing it were concerned. Trevor Walsh, a postgraduate student, wrote a most user-friendly and reliable program. Its one defect was that letters in the word test were not that easy to read which may have resulted in more extensive brain areas than we had intended becoming involved in the test. Electrode placements were always posterior temporal to mid-parietal on both sides.

Another 42 staff in all volunteered. Lo and behold! When doing test (a) they missed fewer target words during left-sided EEG recordings, thus confirming those results from the first experiment that used the same electrode placement. In test (b) they made more errors instead of fewer during left-sided recording, the errors being hits on non-targets instead of target misses.

There were two types of control experiment. One consisted of doing everything as usual except that the EEG pen motors were switched off so that no pen movement could occur. Relay closure, EEG amplifier activity etc. happened as normal. The other type consisted of feeding each pair of EEG leads to all EEG channels instead of having one channel per pair of leads as in the standard experiment. This was done in order to check on the possibility that acoustic feedback from the machine might be causing the results. However, no significant differences in any of the outcome measures were seen during either set of control experiments, strongly suggesting that our positive findings were not due to any electrical or acoustic feedback to subjects.

It may seem from the description so far that the PM paradigm is confirmed, q.e.d. However, this is very far from being the case. The overall probability that the positive findings described above could have been due to chance is around 1 in 500; small enough to be suggestive and interesting but a long way from any 'q.e.d.s'. Also, there was the puzzle over reaction times which, according to the original Penrose collapse hypothesis which was the one we were using, really ought to have been the most sensitive outcome measure but in fact never produced any significant findings. Maybe this was telling us something very interesting about the functions of awareness, but we remained sceptical. Penrose's revised collapse theory *doesn't* suggest that reaction times should be the most sensitive outcome measure, but we didn't know about it at the time.

Overall average reaction times on both the number and the word tests had been about 520 msecs, that on the pattern test about 620 msecs. We wondered if more difficult tests involving longer overall reaction times might produce our hoped-for significant differences. Another 20 volunteers (by this time referred to as 'victims') were found and given both word and pattern tests involving average reaction times in the range 700 to 1400 msecs. The outcome was that all significant differences disappeared from the results! One can make various suggestions about why this was the case which fit in with our hypotheses; for example, perhaps with tests of longer duration there was time for local blood flow changes to occur which performed a similar 'measurement' function to EEG pen movement, but literally outweighed pen movement. However, we had no means of checking on this or other possibilities.

Fatigue was beginning to creep in as all this was still strictly a spare-time activity. It seemed worth making a final effort, though, to ascertain whether looking at different EEG frequency bands would deliver crisper results. We had hitherto amplified as wide a range of frequencies as possible as a catch-all, but this had the side-effect of introducing a lot of electrical noise into the EEG pen movements which might, we speculated, have blurred the results obtained. We abandoned the word test (because of its poor letter quality) and concentrated on a simple pattern test (on which the average reaction time was 590 msecs). The left EEG was set to amplify only in the range 30 to 60 hz, and a variable bandpass filter was installed in the right-sided channel. Another 42 noble victims were tested in groups of seven, using a different right bandpass setting for each group.

The good news in the results was that *individual* subjects often showed significant performance differences; one did not have to rely on summing the results of a batch to find significance as had been necessary previously. The bad news was that the significant performance differences shown by separate individuals were not always in the same direction or on the same outcome measure. There is a statistical method (using binomial probability distributions) for estimating the chances of observing a given number of 'significant' results in a batch of tests. When applied to all the results from all 42 people this method indicated only a 1 in 100 probability that the significant findings could have been there by chance. Target misses were again, as so often previously, the most sensitive measure (the probability of the findings in relation to them being due to chance was less than 1 in 1000). In relation to all three outcome measures, the alpha band results had a 1 in 500 probability of being due to chance, neighbouring bands either 1 in 3 or 1 in 10, and the 35–45 Hz band a 7 out of 10 probability suggesting that there was no experimental effect from it).

Our experiments do in fact suggest that the HE paradigm is inadequate but they lack the unambiguity that we had hoped for. The results can't be taken too seriously unless independent researchers elsewhere confirm them. We suspect that better technical resources than were available to us might help since we got indications that variations in EEG electrode placement in relation to quite small brain areas strongly influenced our results. We had no means of standardising our electrode placement in relation to the brain areas actually being used by individual subjects. Further, it seemed likely that different subjects used different cognitive strategies for task performance and these would need to be controlled in future work. For instance, if some people were using awareness to respond to targets while others were using it to not respond to non-targets, it's hardly surprising that our results should have been so variable however valid the hypotheses. Research, in brief, is best done by full-time professionals.

We have, however, found indications that collapse of a quantum field can influence brain function and that collapse is reflected in EEG activity of around alpha frequency. This is consistent with the PM paradigm, which views awareness as associated in some way with a quantum field, and with earlier evidence about the correlates of alpha activity. There are intriguing hints to be gained about the way in which field collapse influences brain function from its apparent influence on frequency of mistakes, but lack of influence on reaction times. One possible explanation for this is that field collapse influences the chance of some particular thing occupying a global workspace, but cannot affect the speed with which it does so.

'PSI' EXPERIMENTS

The trouble with experiments on telepathy and the like is that they are not usually replicable in the sort of way that scientists like. You can perform two apparently identical experiments and get a significant result from one but zilch from the next. This at once greatly reduces the significance to be attached to the first set of results, so even when parapsychologists report a series of results that are apparently significant overall, critics can always say that other unreported experiments were done elsewhere or elsewhen that mean that the allegedly significant series was simply the result of chance.

Then there are the passions raised on both sides and the accusations of fraud that are hurled about. Such accusations, like those of child sexual abuse now or of witchcraft in the sixteenth century, are easily made and hard to refute not least because they are sometimes justified (some alleged 'witches' really were village charmsters). Some of the fraud is mischievous, some driven by a passion to 'prove' an article of faith which overcomes any desire for intellectual honesty, but most is no different from the practice of all creative scientists who have always been willing to select their findings to fit their theories. This last type of fraud is not due to dishonesty; it is partly a survival stratagem necessary if one is to navigate one's way successfully in a very complex world and partly a result of the fact that it is hard to see or register a fact unless it fits a theory. This sort of thing is normally kept in check by peer review and the like, but where scientists are divided into totally opposed camps it naturally results in acrimony and indignation.

Parapsychologists have thus come to concentrate on seeking low-key but statistically consistent results that are proof against accusations of fraud or sloppiness. They have come very close to success in two areas: telepathy itself and the alleged ability of people to influence random events.

The idea that telepathy can occur has always had its appeal because most people have had occasional experiences that seem to be examples of it, and few believe the (certainly usually and perhaps always correct) statistical account of them. This runs along the lines that, if you have a million people who spend several minutes each day worrying about one another's welfare, it would only be surprising if you did NOT get occasional accounts saying 'I got this terrible feeling that something awful had happened just at the very moment he was run over by a bus'. For a time, forty years ago, the work of Rhine at Duke University apparently confirmed the popular idea and showed that the statistical explanation was not always right, but its reputation has now succumbed to accusations of fraud and statistical sloppiness. One doubts whether conscious fraud occurred, but sloppiness almost certainly crept in as the tests involved were boring to say the least, and must have become mind-numbingly so when carried out, as they were, over more than a decade. However, positive findings from quite rigorously designed experiments have gone on piling up (McCrone, 1993), and it now appears a good deal more likely than not that a weak telepathic faculty does exist.

The evidence that people can weakly influence the output of random number generators is quite good. Radin and Nelson (1989) reviewed over 800 published studies on this topic using meta-analytic techniques and concluded that there is evidence to support the notion of the existence of 'some form of consciousness-related anomaly in random physical systems'. Meta-analysis is in the opinion of some (e.g. Nunn, 1992) a method of distinctly dubious validity. However, it is widely used and accepted in assessing the value of medical treatments so it would seem a little unfair to reject evidence from it in a far less practically important field.

A particularly careful series of experiments has been going on at Princeton since 1979 (Dunne, 1993). People's wishes about outcome appear to have a very weak, but in cumulation highly significant, effect on the output of a variety of physically different types of random number generator. Fascinatingly, two people wishing in concert appear to have slightly more effect than one on his/her own, and there were hints that opposite sex pairs had the most effect, especially if they were married.

How are 'psi' phenomena to be understood assuming, as seems likely, that they do exist? It seems that quantum theory is the front runner in accounting for them. Walker (1984) has given a lengthy review of alternative explanations and, although he does not say so as he is a believer in 'psi', the only one other than quantum theory that appears at all plausible is that they are an illusion. The objection is sometimes raised that telepathy cannot be understood in terms of quantum non-locality because the latter cannot support instantaneous transmission of information. However, this is to misunderstand the nature of telepathy experiments which seek only to ascertain whether correlations of some specified type can occur between people's mental states; any information involved is a later product of the mental state and the success or otherwise of its 'transmission' is something known only to the experimenter. General relativity is therefore not contravened.

Jahn and Dunne (1986) made a detailed analogy between quantum and mental phenomena. Although they state that their comparison is metaphorical only, they go so far as to apply the mathematics of Schrodinger's wave function to mental phenomena, arguing that the individual consciousness is like a single quantum object with probability amplitudes in a 'space' made up of cognition and emotion. They even find analogies in mental life for spin, charge, etc. Paranormal effects, they say, may be due to a derived wave function resulting from putting a subject in an experimental situation where his own wave function will be subsumed in that of the whole set-up. It seems not unreasonable, therefore, to think that evidence for the existence of 'psi' also supports the PM paradigm.

CONCLUSIONS

Though certainty is not to be had, it seems more probable than not that phenomena have been demonstrated which can't be explained on the HE paradigm but which do fit the PM paradigm. This phraseology is undoubtedly cumbersome and cautious, but matches the present state of the evidence. What's the way forward? It appears unlikely that future 'psi' experiments can do much more than confirm earlier results as the effect that they demonstrate is so weak and the effort needed to get reproducible results is so great. Incidentally, the effect on random number generators is far too weak to provide a plausible explanation for the 'Southampton' findings in terms of interference with the randomising apparatus used in it. They may have a role in examining what sorts of co-operation between subjects give rise to the strongest 'psi' phenomena, but otherwise they are likely to be superceded by more objective approaches such as the EEG coherence studies or the Southampton method – or, more likely, a method of the same general type which is so far only a twinkle in someone's eye.

Of course, it may be that the approach advocated by Crick and Koch (1992) will overtake the ones that have been described in more detail. A dark horse worth watching in this connection is the detailed investigation of the effects of anaesthetics on the shape and energy balances of microtubules. Following the ideas of Hameroff (see Chapter 1), there are good reasons for thinking that microtubules might perform basic computations and long-range quantum coherence effects beween them may provide the basis for consciousness. A sufficiently detailed understanding of their behaviour could allow a direct demonstration that he is right (if he is!).

One of the goals set in the introduction was to reach an understanding of what an objective test for the occurrence of awareness might be like. How might Mr Spock's life-form detector actually work? On the PM paradigm, of course, it would be some test (the Southampton one is an example), which could in principle itself be remote, that allowed one to show that a brain activity was subject to non-local influences. It's possible, however, that one does not need the PM paradigm to envisage such a test. Consciousness seems to be especially associated with EEG activities of around alpha frequency and maybe it could be demonstrated that awareness is always accompanied by increased EEG coherence between remote brain areas at these frequencies. I doubt if a test of this sort, though, could ever be carried out from orbit! Any valid test would have very down-to-earth practical applications as well as usefulness in distinguishing truly unconscious from unremembered brain activity. An obvious example is prevention of the rare but horrifying occasions when people thought to be anaesthetised are in fact still conscious.

Although studies of the nature of awareness are at an early stage, encouraging progress has been made. Consciousness is no longer wholly in the domain of philosophers, and there is no reason at all to agree with McGinn (1990) who argued that our brains may be so constituted as never to be able to understand their own capacity for awareness.

REFERENCES

Crick, F. and Koch, C. (1992) 'The Problem of Consciousness', *Scientific American*, September, 111–17.

Dunne, B.J. (1993) 'Co-operator Experiments with an REG Device', in *Cultivating Consciousness*, K.R. Rao (ed.), Praeger: Westport and London.

Grinberg-Zylberbaum, J. and Ramos, J. (1987) 'Patterns of Interhemispheric Correlation During Human Communication', *International Journal of Neuroscience* 36, 41–53.

Jahn, R.G. and Dunne, B.J. (1986) 'On the Quantum Mechanics of Consciousness with Application to Anomalous Phemomena', *Foundations of Physics* 16(8), 721–72.

McCarthy, K. and Goswami, A. (1991) 'Quantum Functionalism and Word-sense Disambiguation Experiments', unpublished paper.

McCrone, J. (1993) 'Roll up for the Telepathy Test', *New Scientist*, 15 May, 29–33.

McGinn, C. (1990) *The Problem of Consciousness: Essays Towards a Resolution*, Basil Blackwell: Oxford.

Nunn, C.M.H. (1992), 'Are Double-blind Controlled Trials Always Necessary?', *Human Psychopharmacology* 7, 55–61.

Nunn, C.M.H., Clarke, C.J.S. and Blott, B.H. (1994) 'Collapse of a Quantum Field May Affect Brain Function', *Journal of Consciousness Studies* 1(1), 127–39.

Orme-Johnson, D., Dillbeck, M.C., Wallace, K.R. and Landrith, G.S. (1982) 'Intersubject EEG Coherence: Is Consciousness a Field?', *International Journal of Neuroscience* 16, 203–9.

Penrose, R. (1989) *The Emperor's New Mind*, Oxford University Press.

Radin, D.L. and Nelson, R.D. (1989) 'Evidence for Consciousness Related Anomalies in Random Physical Systems', *Foundations of Physics* 19(12), 1499–514.

Travis, F.T. and Orme-Johnson, D.W. (1989) 'Field Model of Consciousness: EEG Coherence Changes as Indicators of Field Effects', *International Journal of Neuroscience* 49, 203–11.

Walker, E.H. (1984) 'A Review of Criticisms of the Quantum Mechanical Theory of Psi Phenomena', *Journal of Parapsychology* 48, 277–332.

Woo, C.H. (1981) 'Consciousness and Quantum Interference – an Experimental Approach', *Foundations of Physics* 11, 933–44.

6 Free will, free won't and other topics

As we've now got some clearish ideas and some experimental evidence about what consciousness might actually be like, there are consequences to explore. Does our understanding of awareness fit psychological phenomena which we have either ignored hitherto or mentioned only in passing? Which of our paradigms gives the best fit and do either of them really add to our insights?

Doing this in any very systematic way could be tedious, so it's probably best to pick out topics likely to prove interesting – free will for instance. Hofstadter (1986) does not think much of the notion which simply has no place to lodge in his consciousness paradigm. Like most of us, however, he has a sentimental attachment to the feeling that we possess it, and whimsically reported a friend's comment that, even if we don't have free will, maybe we have free won't (i.e. the ability to freely chose *not* to do something). This is actually a deeper remark than might be thought at first hearing as much brain activity is inhibitory, especially that occurring in the frontal lobes which underpins functions (attention, emotional discriminations, etc.) often associated with awareness. If there's free anything, free won't is likely to happen more often and could even be the sole representative. Of course, it is actually just as unacceptable to the intellectual Hofstadter as free will, except in the trivial sense espoused by Capra (1983: 290) who points out that the more advanced an organism the greater its autonomy in relation to immediate environmental influences.

Sperry (1994), who has made many important contributions to our knowledge of how the brain works and is a supporter of the HE approach, believes that there are two-way interactions between higher level, mentalistic brain functions and lower level neural ones. Control operates in both directions, so mental functions can influence neural happenings; thus, there is an appearance of free will, even though it's not clear what 'free' means in this context. However, as he himself admits, he has no idea what the higher level functions might be that are 'mentalistic', so it is not at all obvious that the apparent free will envisaged by him should be regarded as compatible with the HE paradigm.

An exponent of a variant of the other (PM) paradigm (Squires, 1990) regards the feeling that we have free will as one of the properties of consciousness, though in a sense illusory because in his view we 'choose' all possibilities. Our lives follow mutually inaccessible branchings as a result. Certainly, there is nothing in orthodox quantum theory to support the possibility that real free will exists. The Schrodinger wave function evolves just as deterministically as any Newtonian mechanism and is somewhat more predictable than a classical chaotic system. Agreed, the outcome of wave function collapse is unpredictable, but this happens at random and choice is again excluded. Penrose himself (1989) commented that: 'The vexed question of "free will" hovers at the background throughout this book. . . but it is profound and hard to formulate adequately'. He wonders if it might be related to issues of non-computability.

Marshall (1994) suggests that the capacity for choice, though not necessarily free choice, may arise from the possibility implicit in his wave function collapse theory (see Chapter 3) that collapse is pseudo-random rather than truly random. He thinks that components of the wave function might be semi-conscious in some way, with full consciousness arising as a consequence of collapse. The proposed pseudo-random nature of collapse may allow a preference for a particular semi-conscious possibility to be fully realised. One difficulty with this idea is that wave function collapse is thought by most people to be truly random; another, perhaps greater, problem is that there may be no place within his own paradigm for a concept of consciousness in relation to possibilities still in superposition in the wave function. It's impossible to envisage how they might affect classical neuronal systems without collapsing, and they would have to affect such systems in order to be remembered and so be semi-conscious in the way that he requires. However, this whole system of ideas is still in its infancy, so maybe the problems with Marshall's suggestion are not insuperable.

Like most terms from what philosophers (somewhat patronisingly) tend to call 'folk psychology', free will is not a simple concept. What most of us mean by it most of the time is the capacity to choose between going to the pub, say, or staying in to watch television. If pressed, we would probably agree that choices like this are usually either random or determined by unconscious factors over which we may have no control. Free choice is actually not much in evidence. Then there is the crisis choice: someone who 'chooses' to jump into the raging torrent to save the drowning child instead of prudently going off to seek help. In fact most people who have been in this sort of situation say that they 'just acted', or found themselves acting, and thought about it later. Any role for free choice must be pushed back into the remote past when they turned themselves into the sort of person bound to act heroically instead of with sensible caution – but the choices responsible would mostly have been of the 'Shall I go to the pub?' type, and we have already seen that these may not be free.

There are rare occasions, though, when people do seem to themselves to be genuinely free. These are often associated with difficult choices when there is a lot of psychological pressure: 'Shall I marry John or carry on seeing Andrew?'; 'Shall I whistleblow on my boss or keep my head down?'; 'Shall I take Sylvia off for an illicit weekend or stay faithful to Susie?'. What tends to happen is that a brief moment occurs when all pressure seems to lift and the person feels lucidly free to follow one course or the other; as soon as a choice is made the turmoil tends to come roiling back. Few who have experienced this are inclined to doubt that they have free will, even though it may be truly exercised only once or twice in a lifetime. Are they under an illusion?

The question is of great practical importance as the whole criminal justice system is built on the assumption that people's minds are separable from, and can usually control, their brains. If this assumption is false, one might still wish to punish people to encourage the more widespread occurrence of unfree choices of a type which will make for a law-abiding society. There is something rather 'eighteenth century' about such a policy, though, which does not sit well with modern consciences. In any case, it is probably ineffective (see the endless debates about the effectiveness or otherwise of capital punishment as a deterrent). Moving on to nineteenth-century ideas, particularly Marxism, one might say that people's behaviour clearly is unfree but society requires protection from those unlucky enough to have been impelled into antisocial behaviours; hence punishment is not appropriate, but the gulags are!

Peter Fenwick (1993) has pointed out that behaviour, including criminal behaviour, can be described by 'mind words' or by 'brain words'. People may have guilty intentions or they may have epileptic automatisms; they may be irritable and selfish or they may have low serotonin levels in brain-stem nuclei. When it can be shown through the use of objective tests such as EEG or brain scanning that brain words are the most appropriate ones to use in connection with a piece of behaviour, people should not be regarded as having criminal responsibility for it. He concludes:

> As knowledge of brain functioning increases and imaging facilities become more available, it will become easier to detect minor degrees of brain malfunction, and the usefulness of the concept of *mens rea*, the guilty mind, may diminish even further.

However, it rather looks from what has been said so far as though *all* words used about behaviour should be brain words, as mind words are either surrogates for more accurate brain words or are meaningless. Clearly, it would be silly to try to translate the whole language of psychology into brain words (trying to do so would be to commit the philosophical sin of making a category mistake), but it is valid to infer that one should attempt translation of mind words relevant to the immediate antecedents of behaviour. The mind word 'choose', for instance, should, in relation to actions chosen, properly refer to the outcome of various neuronal happenings associated with an illusory feeling that the brain self-model could have selected a different outcome. This seems to be an inescapable consequence of the HE paradigm on which there is nothing going on in the brain other than neuronal events of an unpredictable but nevertheless entirely deterministic nature.

It's possible that the PM paradigm offers a loophole which would restore meaning to the concept of free will in relation to action. Readers will probably already have noticed that it reintroduces a sort of dualism by the back door. There is the classical neuronal activity involving depolarisation waves and synaptic transmission, and there are the apparently secondary Bose–Einstein condensates or whatever which underlie awareness. The point is that the quantum phenomena are not entirely determined by the classical nervous activity for two reasons; first, the classical activity can only increase the chance that a particular quantum state will manifest itself; second, and more important in the present context, the quantum state has a different, more direct, relationship to the external world from the classical activity. Information in classical neuronal systems is dealt with in mappings and symbolisms which have an at-arms-length relationship to everything outside themselves, while that in the quantum state enfolds, so to speak, its sources including those in the outside world. For these reasons, although awareness can be regarded as usually faithfully reflecting some aspect of current neuronal activity, it may sometimes be slightly or even markedly different.

This potential difference in information content would be of academic interest only if the quantum state cannot influence the classical system since actions would still be wholly determined by classical neuronal goings-on regardless of the content of consciousness. However, there is quite strong circumstantial evidence that awareness can do things, constrained though it may be by Libet's findings (see Chapter 2). There is folk psychology again which probably overstates the case in regarding consciousness as the main source of actions and decisions, but should not be entirely dismissed. There is the Darwinian argument to the effect that awareness appears to have been selected for in the course of evolution, but is probably energetically costly, so must have some function important to survival. Then there is the (weak) experimental evidence which suggests that it is efficacious and might influence the probability of some particular set of neural activity coming to occupy a brain 'global workspace'.

Suppose that classical nervous activity favoured one candidate for entry to a global workspace while the quantum state favoured another, the result could surely amount to our common experience of wanting to do or think something, often finding that we had actually done something else, but nevertheless sometimes following our conscious intention. Both the classical system and the quantum state follow their own laws in which free choice has no place, but just possibly something very like it emerges from the interactions between the two. Perhaps, in some rather limited sense, the quantum system can monitor the classical one and attempt to bring it into line when necessary – or make it go off the rails if it is the quantum system that is misbehaving.

One may think from this that criminal lawyers should be rooting for the PM paradigm. Certainly the concepts of criminal responsibility and of punishment seem more appropriate in relation to an inherently aware system which probably has some limited autonomy than to the puppet of brain machinery implied by the HE paradigm. Should one, however, punish PM paradigm awareness for following its own laws willy nilly, or for failing in the uncertain task of imposing itself on brain machinery? Readers are welcome to try to decide!

ATTENTION

This most natural-seeming of abilities presents some difficulties from the conceptual point of view, partly because it is not unitary and partly because it moulds the form of successive qualia but also enters them (there is a subjective 'feel' of what it is like to be paying attention). Although it forms part of the ordinary stream of awareness, it appears to exist in a different time-frame and to have a controlling role. Can it be reconciled with either or both of our paradigms?

William James, the very influential late nineteenth-century psychologist and brother of Henry James the novelist, distinguished between automatic attention, such as is involved in riding a bicycle once one has fully learned the skill, and conscious, voluntary attention (James, 1950 [late nineteenth century]). Only the latter is relevant here, but it's worth noting that the adjectives 'conscious' and 'voluntary' are independent in that they may not both apply at the same time. For instance, a daydreaming cycle-rider has little choice about what will next enter his awareness if he gets a puncture, nor has a mother whose baby starts to cry. The other side of the coin is familiar to crossword addicts who get stuck on a clue; a solution will often pop up if they banish the clue from consciousness for a time, yet voluntary attention to it of some sort must have continued so that the brain could go on dealing with it.

The fact that attention can both be a component of qualia and determine their content is like an upside-down version of the apparent paradox concerning how the specious present can contain information about a sequence of notes within it. The 'units' on which attention works are presumably the 100 msecs, seven item ones discussed in Chapter 2. The neuronal activity subserving attention no doubt endures for a lot more than 100 msecs in most circumstances, but this would not prevent it from contributing to one or more of the seven items within each moment of awareness, so there is not really any paradox in this case either.

There is, of course, a controller further up the hierarchy than attention itself. Emotion in all its forms fills this role. Think how difficult it is to ignore the smell of food when you are hungry. At a more sophisticated level, it is presumably the emotion of curiosity that made you read this book.

In short, attention is evidently simply yet another complex brain mechanism subserved by machines involving cortex and brain stem that run on dopamine in at least part of their circuitry (Matthysse, 1978). Only a proportion of its total activity is conscious, and which of its activities shall enter awareness seems to vary with circumstances. Therefore, it fits in naturally with either of our paradigms, provided the HE one is stretched a little to include a global workspace type of concept. No paradoxes are involved since its relationship to awareness is no different in principle from that of perception, cognition and so forth.

SLEEP, DREAMS AND HALLUCINATIONS

While no one knows why we sleep, one of its most obvious characteristics is loss of the ability to pay sustained, voluntary attention to anything. This statement, however, needs quite a bit of qualification. Sustained, and at least partly wished, attention can continue throughout sleep, witness again the new mother and her crying baby which will wake her a lot faster than anything else. Then there is the rare condition of lucid dreaming in which the dreamer is aware of his state and can sometimes to a limited extent direct the course of his dream. It's probably truer to say that, during sleep, the faculty of voluntary attention is down-regulated to a very marked extent. There are neural machines in the brain stem for doing this, just as there are machines for inducing paralysis of all muscles (except those used for breathing and eye movements) during REM sleep. It's worth adding in parenthesis that of course the word 'voluntary' is not being used, either in this section or in the previous one on attention, to imply the existence of free will but merely the subjective feeling of being able to choose one's focus of attention.

Then there are the famous two phases of sleep – slow wave and REM. During the latter cortical energy use is high and vivid dreams occur. Dreaming of this type can thus be considered a flow of awareness relatively unconstrained by attention as well as perception (slow wave sleep dreams are no doubt significantly modified by a relatively low cortical energy use which is more likely to be due to some brain mechanism than to be a consequence of the low key nature of the dreams themselves). It's worth dwelling a little on three of the qualities shown by REM dreams; their capriciousness, the habitual unconcern of dreamers to inconsistencies in their experience and the fact that dreams often seem entirely real for as long as they last.

Their capriciousness fits neatly with our image of awareness as a butterfly flitting over the brain quilt. Without attention or a consistent input from the external world to guide it, it is even freer than usual to settle momentarily where the impulse takes it. Of course, the more accurate, if less appealing, picture should be of neural events jostling to gain entry to a sort of arena of awareness and doing so more or less at random in the absence of consistent influences from attentional mechanisms or the outside world. There is nothing in this to give pause to either of our paradigms.

That it can seem entirely natural to a dreamer to find that he has suddenly shrunk to the size of a mouse for instance, like Alice in Wonderland, is (as Alice would have said) 'curiouser'. Unconcern like this is not uncommon after physical damage to brain association areas when people can 'forget about' the whole of one side of their body or be unaware that they are unable to see. Presumably what is happening in dreams is that the relevant association areas are sometimes not activated or not entering awareness as they normally would. This does actually pose some, relatively minor, problems for the HE approach in which neuronal groups, if sufficiently activated to occupy the stage of awareness, should function as wholes carrying along their usual associations. One would have to bring in an additional argument to the effect that lack of attentional or perceptual inputs weakens the cohesiveness of groups and so allows them to occupy awareness in fragmented forms.

The subjective realism often possessed by dreams appears, on the other hand, to cause problems for PM ideas. It was argued that the subjective essence of experience derives from quantum events in the brain enfolding the realities of the outside world, so how could dreams share a similar essence? Surely their occurrence refutes the PM interpretation. Actually, this is less of a problem than might be supposed because there's no time limit on some quantum non-locality effects, and it's by no means clear what the time constraints are on the bulk of non-local entanglements. Even when awake, our experience is always around half a second behind the time and so is always mediated through memory of a sort. The more remote in time the memory, the less vivid (except in certain rare circumstances such as abreaction or Proustian recall) an experience of it will seem, perhaps because the amount of available neural detail fades with time. But when there is no current input, as when one is asleep, it is reasonable to assume that remoter memories when activated will acquire a relative subjective immediacy. Dreaming can thus be considered an experience of haphazard memory-based neural activity consistent with a PM view or an HE one.

Hallucinations provide another instance of a divorce between experience and present reality. Some of them (those occurring in deliria or some intoxications) can in all likelihood be understood as waking dreams in which memory-like records have become so strongly activated as to appear as vivid or more so than 'present' experience. In temporal lobe epilepsy, a particular neural engram based experience can fire off so to speak and entirely replace for brief periods experience of the outside world. In delirium tremens, the insects and snakes are usually to be seen crawling over real surfaces.

Other hallucinations (the 'voices' of schizophrenics, for instance) may in a sense be the opposite of dreams in that they may originate from overactive automatic attention instead of being associated with reduced attention. However, the outcome may often be similar in that any inappropriate increased attention can result in overactivation of old engrams relative to current perceptual inputs (see, for example, Elkins *et al.*, 1991 or Myles-Worsley *et al.*, 1991). It looks, therefore, as if both our paradigms can accommodate all these phenomena.

UNDERSTANDING

Academic debate over whether 'understanding' is a sub-category of information processing or something quite different has tended to centre around Searle's (1980) famous Chinese room argument. He pictured a room containing a man who knew no Chinese and a complicated book of rules, written in the man's own language, for transforming one set of Chinese characters into another. Chinese people would write questions and post them into the room, the man would consult his rule book, deduce a suitable reply, draw it and post it back out. Because it was a very comprehensive and reliable rule book, the Chinese people always got sensible replies. To them it would look as if the room understood their questions but clearly, said Searle, although information was being processed there was no understanding anywhere in the system. Therefore, understanding is different from information processing q.e.d.

On the whole, opinion has tended to support Searle's conclusion. The most convincing objection is that the system as a whole, man and rule book together, *did* possess understanding; the appearance to the contrary being simply a result of the fact that we are not used to seeing the internal workings that lead to understanding. If we could peer inside our brains all we would find would be a whole set of sub-systems to no individual member of which could understanding be attributed. As there appears to be no logically watertight way of refuting this objection, it is interesting that Searle's argument should have continued to gain support for as much as a decade. It's probably because everyone has a gut feeling that the two are different and would like to be convinced: folk psychology again!

The distinction that needs explanation can be illustrated by thinking about what is meant by understanding a foreign language from a different angle to that used by Searle. I speak a smattering of French and consider that I understand the word '*avec*' because I don't need to translate it to know that it has some of the same meanings as 'with'; it directly conveys an awareness of togetherness. On the other hand, although I know that the word '*fleuve*' means 'river', I have first to translate it to get any sense of riverness from it. I do not really understand *fleuve*. Or think back to maths lessons at school and meeting the sign '='. It didn't take long to get to handle it in the right way, but reaching a stage at which it triggered automatic understanding that the thing on the left of the sign was equivalent to the thing on the right probably took a lot longer.

Is the difference, then, to be found in the complexity of the associations called up by an item? Understanding takes time to develop because it takes time to acquire the necessary richness of association. Well, no; this does not suffice as an explanation. Think, this time, of solving a crossword clue. When you *don't* understand it you are calling up all sorts of associations but when you do get it, it at once simplifies and leaps out at you, so to speak.

The difference between understanding and information processing is that the former entails conscious apprehension of an essence of whatever is being understood whereas information processing need not be conscious and, when it is, lacks the immediacy of understanding even though the conclusions reached may be just as accurate. How do our two paradigms deal with this difference?

HE ideas have to agree with the major objection to the Chinese room argument. On them, understanding is a sub-category of information processing distinguished from the general run sometimes by complexity or perhaps sometimes by where it is carried out in the brain. Overt understanding (as opposed to implicit, latent understanding) is simply the word for the outcomes of information processing that become conscious as a result of entering a global workspace or whatever.

The PM account is quite different; understanding is what happens when the relevant quantum processes in the brain enfold an aspect of the real world. It is the cognitive counterpart of perceiving a quality such as blueness. In relation to comprehending a word in French, it can be regarded as involving the formation of a non-local relationship with the French language as instantiated in the brains of French speakers that one has met or recorded in various media that one has come across. In relation to understanding a crossword clue, it involves collapse of a wave function following computation of a good 'fit' with the clue. Although only possible when based on a groundwork of neural information processing, the onset of understanding represents a discontinuity analogous to crystallisation or, more accurately, the onset of superfluidity when a liquid is cooled below a critical temperature. To some this account will seem more psychologically true than the HE one, to others simply far fetched. Either way, it is certainly more interesting than the HE story.

BEAUTY

> The fowls of the air abide shall and dwell,
> Who moved by nature to hop here and there,
> Among the green branches their songs shall excel.
>
> (W. Kethe, from his rendering of Psalm CIV)

> The mind is its own place, and in itself
> Can make a heav'n of hell, a hell of heav'n.
> What matter where, if I be still the same,
>
> (John Milton, *Paradise Lost*)

Almost all would agree that the first quotation is ugly and the second beautiful. Not only the banality of sentiment and clumsiness of expression in the first make it jar; even a non-English speaker, one suspects, would dislike its rhythmic and consonantal properties. What gives Milton the opposite of these qualities is harder to pin down. This is not the place to indulge in literary criticism at any length, but there is clearly a puzzle over what aesthetic terms might represent in neurological reality; over how to translate the language of art into mind/brain words.

The static visual arts (painting, sculpture, etc.) are the easiest exemplars to cope with as they leave out a dimension, time, with which it is notoriously difficult to deal. Gombrich (1982) has forcefully pointed out that a picture, say, cannot be distinguished from a piece of music on grounds of the time needed to appreciate it because as many moments are needed to scan a painting as to listen to a musical phrase. All the same music, or cinema for that matter, depend in an essential way on formal temporal structures which are either absent or much less important in the static arts. Painting alone poses problems enough. Ample goddesses by Reubens can give enormous pleasure, but so can Francis Bacon's revolting pictures of people as slabs of decaying meat – and the core of the delight to be derived from these superficially very different artists is, many would say, *the same*.

Could it all be due to inbuilt circuitry? Obviously people are genetically predisposed, to varying degrees, to seeing snakes and spiders as horrible, though *afficionados* of both find beauty in them. Some interesting studies have been done on what makes for a beautiful female face. The first answer to be given (Symons, 1979) was 'averageness'. Symons took a whole lot of photos of individual women's faces and extracted one composite image from them. The composite was judged more attractive than any of the photos of real women. However, he turns out to have been not quite right. Perrett *et al.* (1994) got people to select attractive faces from a bunch of pictures, then made composites of the ones selected as well as of the whole bunch. The composite made from photos assessed as individually attractive was rated more beautiful than the composite derived from the whole group; further, the more attractive composite differed from the other in exactly the same respects when the procedure was repeated in two different cultures (Japanese and English). It looks, therefore, as if cultural factors do not influence ratings of female beauty. The researchers think the ratings might be to do with pre-programmed estimates of fertility potential or perhaps of 'cuteness' related to the known human preference for baby-like appearance with big eyes.

Nature in the form of neural pre-programming, then, can probably influence aesthetic judgements. No doubt nurture can do the same. People who have a lot to do with horses, for instance, are often willing to pay good money for the most drab and stilted-looking pictures of eighteenth-century hunters and hacks. Country gents seem able to find a beauty in paintings of dead pheasants which escapes the rest of us. Education and familiarity also play a part; Picasso's famous *Guernica*, dominated as it is by a caricature of a startled horse's head, appears grotesquely ugly at first sight yet one can learn to see beauties in it. To allow all this does not really help to solve the puzzle.

Abstract painting, being the 'purest' type, may be the easiest to understand. Bridget Riley is one of our leading abstract artists. Dougary (1994) wrote about her:

> So what, precisely, is she trying to do? In the swirling movement of the lines of her earlier work, or the hypnotic rhythm of her more recent bands of colour, she is not merely attempting to convey, say, the sparkle on the water, or the flowing movement of a curtain rippled by the breeze. Riley is after the thing itself. The very essence of 'sparkle-ness'. . . the essence of 'flowing-ness'. . . [This], of the many different readings of her work, strikes me as right – however clumsy it sounds. It is the only one which sufficiently conveys the sense in which Riley's paintings are a bonding of the intellect, the essence of the idea of a thing, and the senses, the physical experience of being drawn into that element.

This passage, of course, has strong resonances with our PM view of awareness. Dougary might as well have said that Riley tries to put on canvas for others to see the quantum objects created in her brain by certain experiences. Perhaps all artists try to do this and we honour them so much, when they are successful, because they show us what the essence of our own awareness is like or could be like. Aesthetic pleasure may be the outcome both of the artist's success in representing her own Bose condensates and their degree of congruence with our habitual ones. An unsuccessful artist would be seen as false, shallow or trite, while a successful one too different from ourselves could be seen as jarring or hideous. Subjective beauty would be an intrinsic quality of the quantum objects whose shape is dependent on nature, nurture and education. Some shapes, those conforming to the golden rule, for instance, would have it, others not. This formulation probably carries an implication that ideal, Platonic beauty also exists, but that is something for artists and philosophers to debate; we are already straying quite a way beyond the scope of this book.

Is there an HE interpretation? Certainly something could be cobbled together about how paintings of the right sort, when processed through a range of cortical maps, trigger pleasurable associations and memories because their representations happen to use the right neurones to do so, and this is felt as aesthetic pleasure or a sense of beauty. Any such account, however, might be thought itself to lack the quality allegedly accounted for. It is thus amusing mainly because it tends to unravel the subtext of the type of argument that Hofstadter might have used for proposing it in the first place!

CONCLUSIONS

Both of our paradigms can accommodate or explain the phenomena mentioned in this Chapter but, except in relation to attention, there is a marked contrast in the quality of explanation given, PM ideas illuminate their subject and stretch the imagination; HE ones are dismissive of everyday insights, of folk psychology, and require that one should often attempt to confine all sorts of fascinating realms of thought and experience within the dour rigidities of 'brain words'. Is this analogous to the contrast that a nineteenth-century biologist might have seen between the concept of vital force (standing in for PM ideas) and Mendelian genetics (for HE ideas)? Mendelism, of course, turned out to be basically correct and eventually led to the marvels of molecular biology, while *élan vital* has sunk without trace except as a dated phrase divorced from biological theory.

This analogy is actually not a very good one since we, with our privileged access to our own awareness, are in a somewhat different situation from biologists studying external phenomena. Of course, looked at via a PM perspective, the two situations are not so different as one might suppose, but they are still not exactly the same. Folk psychology has a validity not necessarily possessed by folk biology. Paradoxically enough, folk psychology would appear to have greater relative validity in terms of HE ideas, with which it does not fit at all well, as the relation between external phenomena and awareness is less close according to them. Then PM ideas, unlike the concept of *élan vital*, derive from the deepest truths concerning the nature of the physical universe of which we are aware. Further, it has to be remembered that such experimental evidence as there is, recounted in the last Chapter, favours the PM paradigm. For all these reasons, but especially because it is so much more interesting from the point of view of all but a few neural network specialists, we shall drop His Excellency in the next Chapter and concentrate on looking at further consequences of PM ideas, though we've not seen the last of the former as far as the rest of the book is concerned.

REFERENCES

Capra, F. (1983) *The Turning Point: Science, Society and the Rising Culture*, Flamingo: London.

Dougary, G. (1994) 'Between the Lines', *Times Magazine*, 5 March, 8–12.

Elkins, I.J., Cromwell, R.L. and Asarnow, R.F. (1991) 'Span of Apprehension in Schizophrenic Patients as a Function of Distractor Masking and Laterality', *Journal of Abnormal Psychology* 101, 53–60.

Fenwick, P. (1993) 'Brain, Mind and Behaviour: Some Medico-legal Aspects', *British Journal of Psychiatry* 163, 565–73.

Gombrich, E.H. (1982) 'Moment and Movement in Art', in *The Enigma of Time*, P.T. Landberg (ed.), Adam Hilger: Bristol.

Hofstadter, D.R. (1986) *Metamagical Themas*, Penguin Books: Harmondsworth.

James, W. (1950) [late nineteenth century] *Principles of Psychology*, Dover: New York.

Marshall, I.N. (1994) 'Three Kinds of Thinking', paper given at conference 'Towards a Scientific Basis for Consciousness', to be published by MIT Press Boston.

Matthysse, S. (1978) 'A Theory of the Relation between Dopamine and Attention', *Journal of Psychiatric Research* 14, 241–8.

Myles-Worsley, M., Johnston, W.A. and Wender, P.H. (1991) 'Spontaneous Selective Attention in Schizophrenia', *Psychiatry Research* 39, 167–79.

Penrose, R. (1989) *The Emperor's New Mind*, Oxford University Press.

Perrett, D.I., May, K.A. and Yoshikawa, S. (1994) 'Facial Shape and Judgements of Female Attractiveness', *Nature* 368, 239–42.

Searle, J.R. (1980) 'Minds, Brains and Programs', *Behavioural and Brain Sciences* 3, 417–57.

Sperry, R.W. (1994) 'Holding Course Amid Shifting Paradigms', in *New Metaphysical Foundations of Modern Science*, W. Harman and J. Clark (eds), Institute of Noetic Sciences, California.

Squires, E. (1990) *Conscious Mind in the Physical World*, Adam Hilger: Bristol.

Symons, D. (1979) *The Evolution of Human Sexuality*, Oxford University Press.

7 The functions of awareness

Many writers on this theme flounder a bit since, as has been remarked previously, no one actually knows for certain what consciousness does or what it is for. A commonly used strategy is to propose some favourite theory about its functions and centre discussion around that. The plan here is a variation on this method. Some of the approaches used by others will be mentioned and examined in the context of the PM paradigm to see what, if any, light it throws on them. Perhaps PM theory will prove a sufficiently sturdy prop to prevent too much floundering.

BIOLOGICAL PERSPECTIVES

Most writers who use this approach at all seem agreed that consciousness evolved and that we share some recognisable form of it with at least the higher animals. Dawkins (1993) (Marian Dawkins, that is, not the better known Richard Dawkins who wrote *Blind Watchmaker* and would, one suspects, avoid any discussion of awareness like the plague!), is a particularly eloquent exponent of this view. As always happens there are dissenting voices; for instance Jaynes (1990) who wrote a stimulating and enjoyable, but arguably somewhat eccentric, book claiming that consciousness started around 4000 BC, so reminding one of Archbishop Ussher and his famous calculation from the Old Testament that the creation must have occurred in 4004 BC.

If it is accepted that awareness evolved, attention can be centred on what its earliest forms must have been like and how it developed from them, or on what Darwinian advantage it might provide. The latter approach is over rather uncertain ground as there seems to be no inherent reason why it should not be the ineffective epiphenomenon of something else that does provide advantage. People following this line, therefore, tend to argue that their particular idea involves consciousness in some essential way. Luckily, as has been contended earlier in this book, the PM approach frees us from all but the most lingering of fears that awareness might actually do nothing.

An example of the first strategy is Humphrey's (1992) proposal that the origins of awareness are to be found in simple organisms' responses to stimulation of their surfaces in the form of feedback to said surfaces. When they evolve into more sophisticated creatures the 'surfaces' are internalised to become perceptual cortex in their brains and feedback to this from 'feeling' areas of their brains produces consciousness according to the HE paradigm. An idea of the same general type, which might be considered more plausible than Humphrey's, is due to Newman (1994). He suggests that the most primitive form of consciousness is an expression of the self-model which becomes necessary as soon as a brain has evolved sufficiently to include maps of its surroundings. Without a representation of the position of the self, such maps would of course be useless. He also makes the intriguing suggestion that the primitive self-model in question is simply the zero co-ordinates in spatial maps; a simplification with a touch of genius in it.

Ideas like this are interesting in relation to how neural functions may have evolved, but in PM terms they can have nothing directly to do with the development of consciousness. However, it is implicit in the ideas of both Frohlich and Hameroff (see Chapters 1 and 4) that the mechanism for producing consciousness is present in all cells (Frohlich) or in all cells that contain microtubules, particularly animal ones (Hameroff). A sort of proto-awareness therefore existed right from the earliest stages of evolution, though of course self-consciousness of the sort that we have to endure would have been a much later development dependent on the evolution of sufficiently elaborate neural machinery.

Humphrey (1986) also had a go at the Darwinian approach and suggested that the selective advantage which gave rise to consciousness was that it allows prediction of how one's neighbour is likely to behave. Certainly, for social creatures, members of the same species can provide more of an opportunity or a threat than anything else in their environments. It is reasonable to suppose that a clear picture of oneself is useful in predicting what one would do in someone else's shoes, and this ability can save all sorts of unpleasantness. The idea probably correctly identifies one of the drives behind the evolution of larger brains, but strains to account for awareness as such. It's much more comfortable to think that awareness evolved in elaboration along with brains but there was never a moment when a particular brain mechanism developed somehow to switch on consciousness.

If Penrose's specific collapse theory (see Chapter 3) is correct there may have been a sort of rheostat turning up, so to speak, awareness over the course of evolution. This applies most clearly with the 1989 version of his theory; the more recent version predicts a similar effect, but in relation to a smaller brain size than would be supposed on his earlier ideas. Very small brains may lack the intrinsic (superpositional) mass differences necessary to collapse the wave function, so Bose condensates in them are a *post hoc* occurrence dependent on the consequences of behaviour (i.e. wave function collapse won't occur until the organism has moved to the left, say, instead of the right). As brains got bigger, their intrinsic activity ever more readily exceeded the Penrose criterion for collapse (or rapid collapse on the new version), so awareness occurred at an ever earlier stage in connection with any particular piece of neural activity. Libet (Chapter 2) has shown that it takes up to half a second for us to become aware of something, and a brain using many fewer neurones than we do in some specific connection might take a lot longer to achieve consciousness. Moreover, small brains could take a very long time indeed to be aware of purely intrinsic activity, such as cogitation, that never becomes correlated with events having appreciable mass effects.

There's one possible way round this restriction on awareness in small brains, namely to base it on long-range coherence effects involving separate organisms. It has been seriously proposed (by van der Post, 1962) that this is precisely what termites do, though at the time he lacked any adequate theory to back up his suggestion. The individual white ant is no more conscious that one of our neurones, he said, but the whole colony does have an awareness. Hofstadter, of course, proposed the same thing (see pp. 62–3) but it was only a parable to him; he probably never dreamed that it might be an actuality.

The conclusion we are left with, whether or not Penrose's collapse theory is correct, is that proto-consciousness was always there. There never was a time when some sophisticated awareness suddenly materialised like Athena leaping fully armed from the head of Zeus. If trying to imagine what the most primitive awareness was like, picturing automatically reaching out a hand to catch a ball and then subsequently noticing that one's hand had got a ball in it might not be too far off the mark; except of course that it is impossible for us to ever fully turn off associative memory which would not have been a feature of the primitive state. The PM view thus turns most interpretations, though not that reached by Humphrey six years after his first try, on their heads in that it sees awareness as a primal phenomenon which bided its time until it could come into its own, while other brain activities are the latecomers.

There is still at least one puzzle remaining from the point of view of neural evolution over the last 100 million years or more! That is, why was awareness incorporated in these new-fangled brains, so demonstrably more efficient than consciousness itself at processing the large amounts of information needed for survival in a world growing ever more complex? Is it that awareness cannot be divorced from living cells or, as seems more likely, is it somehow of help to brains? Maybe there are creatures in whom brains do function without awareness, living automata. Approaches other than purely biological ones are needed to decide whether consciousness might be a help or a hindrance (or neutral) to creatures like ourselves.

WHAT MIGHT AWARENESS DO FOR THE BRAIN?

This question would be thought nonsensical by many brain scientists or, as a philosopher might put it in an apparently restrained but really more damning way, ill posed. They tend to ask the quite different question: 'What necessary brain function can I think of that might plausibly engender consciousness?'. The self-model is one such which has appealed to many thinkers including Newman; another favourite candidate is the 'supervisor' which may be necessary in massively parallel computing systems like the brain to unscramble log jams of information which have a good chance of building up (see, for example, Hundert, 1987). A third is the global workspace which has proved a most useful concept since we first met it in Chapter 4, though in PM terms it is of course insufficient on its own to account for our butterfly.

The claim made here is that it's in fact sensible to ask what awareness does for the brain, since brains appear to have gone out of their way over the course of evolution to nurture it. On the other hand it's not so sensible to ask how particular brain mechanisms might engender consciousness because most cells have the potential to provide a basis for it and the role of brain mechanisms is limited to moulding it into evermore elaborate forms.

There is a necessary preliminary. Namely, to ask whether there is any plausible means by which awareness could affect the brain. In an outline sort of way, one can see that there is. The Bose–Einstein condensates which comprise awareness on the PM view are unique lowest energy states of whatever system they involve. When they materialise, a redistribution of some of the energy within the brain will result and when they decay the situation will be reversed. Most of the energy involved will be thermal (heat), but it's likely that some will be electrical. Local temperature changes alone could have an effect on the function of classical neuronal systems, but of course any electrical changes will have a more powerful and direct effect. It is, therefore, safe to say that the occurrence of condensates is likely to have quite major effects on classical brain functions, even though quantitative estimates can't be made because there is no information about detail. Penrose (1994) has speculated that there may be a specific chain of causation in which Bose condensates affect microtubular computations which in turn affect the structure or activity of nerve cell synapses.

This digression gives the original question (what might awareness do for the brain?) some added force as it seems that awareness not only uses energy, because local temperature changes will overall dissipate heat energy, a commodity not readily squandered by successful competitors in the Darwinian arena, but its occurrence also tends to alter patterns of ordinary nervous activity in an inherently unpredictable way. It looks superficially to be an unmitigated nuisance that should have been eliminated from well-ordered brains at the first evolutionary opportunity. Yet it has persisted and even flourished. This is certainly not because it seems to aid information handling in a quantitative way; as we've already seen it does the opposite. Crossword addicts tend not to think much of its qualitative value either – unconscious processes often appear better from their point of view!

Awareness must carry considerable benefits to outweigh these disadvantages. Possible benefits can be looked at from two angles. First, is the Penrose one which can be thought of as regarding consciousness as an expression of the stopping criterion for quantum computations. This sort of computation might be of great advantage to small brains with few physically separate parallel channels (even though, on Penrose's earlier collapse theory, they could rarely benefit from such an advantage). We have so many parallel channels that it's not obvious that having quantum superpositions as well would help much. Marcel (see Chapter 1) showed that information is already subject to every conceivable manipulation, so far as can be seen, before awareness gets to grips with it. But could Marcel's results relate to possibilities in superposition rather than those in physically separate channels? This actually seems very unlikely because there is probably no way in which components of a wave function could affect subsequent neuronal behaviour without collapsing, but Marcel showed that behaviour is influenced by parallel computations.

The trouble with parallel systems, of course, is that they can produce parallel answers; for instance, 'That patch of shadow over there is dappled because of the sun shining through the leaves' and 'That patch of shadow over there is dappled because of the spots on the skin of the leopard that's hiding there'. As we've seen already, quantum computation can arrive at approximately correct answers faster than classical computation so there may well be advantage in following both methods and taking the result of the quantum one as a basis for action when the classical parallel system gives conflicting answers. This is similar to the idea mentioned earlier that awareness is an expression of the activity of a sort of overseer of brain activity; maybe it can, among much else, express the function of not so much an overseer as a referee, and it's this ability which is responsible for Darwinian fitness.

The other angle leads to much the same conclusion as the first, but in a rather stronger form. Classical neuronal systems rely on indirect feedback from the environment in order to learn whether or not their interpretations and conclusions are correct. Education by parents or other members of a social group can short-circuit this process to some extent, but is not infallible even in our societies, let alone those of animals. Sometimes the feedback will be of a fatal sort, so any way of gaining direct apprehension of the nature of what is encountered in the world would be very helpful. This is just what awareness does; it will be remembered that brain quantum objects representing aspects of the world are, in a much stronger sense than neuronal mappings, interwoven with those aspects. To uneducated neurones in the visual cortex the pattern made by seeing a lion's claws will be just a pattern, but in awareness it will carry a sense of sharpness; it may even be not too far-fetched to envisage a direct apprehension of grasping and tearing very useful to naïve prey.

The answer to our question appears to be that awareness helps the brain to promote survival by achieving, in certain situations that may sometimes be critical, a more accurate comprehension of the external world than is available to classical neuronal systems, through improved computation and more direct apprehension. It would be nice to be able to specify precisely how it gets its message across to the classical systems, but at present one can only utter generalities about how it is likely to do so through effects on attention and the inhibition or facilitation of action, mediated perhaps in a global workspace; effects that have co-evolved with the classical systems over millions of years.

The benefits of awareness have come with a huge price tag: the pain and suffering of countless generations of sentient creatures. Brains on their own could have shown avoidance behaviour and stress reactions but they would not have brought the experience of distress into the world. Of course, there have been benefits too – love, joy, the experience of beauty – but it would take a very determined Dr Pangloss ('All's for the best in the best of all possible worlds') to maintain that the cost has not been overwhelming. It is likely, also, that there are other costs and other benefits still to be considered.

THE 'QUANTUM SOCIETY' REVISITED

Doris Lessing, a mistress of English prose and of dispassionate observation of human foibles, has written (among much else) a series of five science fiction books under the generic title *Canopus in Argos*. Their theme centres around questions of how groups of people are linked, where fashions come from, what influences the growth of societies or determines the onset of attacks of barbarism. She has some delightful interpolated concepts; for instance, the hospital for rhetorical diseases (an institution badly needed for the treatment of many health service personnel at present!) pictured in her book entitled *Sentimental Agents in the Volyen Empire*. The first stage of treatment consisted of putting people in a ward with huge plate glass windows, perched on a cliff above a stormy ocean with a darkling forest in the background, while playing to them continuous tapes of Tschaikowsky and Wagner. The idea was that they would soon sicken of turbulent emotion and want nothing more than a diet of cool reason and, perhaps, a nice cup of tea.

Her overall conclusions are rather traditional. They seem to be that people are subsumed into groups, subject to group laws, which determine to some extent individual actions and even what range of thoughts it is possible to think. All this is influenced by ill-understood forces of good and evil. Any folk psychologist who has seen how the tribes of Yugoslavia or Central Africa seem impelled to behave nowadays just like Vandals, Goths or Lombards in the fifth and sixth centuries must agree. The modern tribes are perhaps a bit more lethal, but that is probably because they have access to better technology which they manage to use without any apparent influence on their underlying mind-sets. Fashions in disease comprise a more accessible example of mass behaviours apparently beyond the control of many individuals, but this will be saved for the next Chapter.

Confronted with phenomena like these, people's usual reaction is to say that they are the outcome of 'laws' of psychology and sociology which are at present, it must be admitted, poorly understood. The laws in question are conceived as analogous to Newton's laws of motion. Zohar and Marshall (1993), using of course the PM paradigm, pointed out at length that mental laws are not very like Newtonian ones. They are more analogous to the mathematics of the wave function where everything is indeterminate until some specific 'measurement' is made. Further, there will be non-local correlations between individual minds dependent on the closeness of their previous associations. They develop an optimistic view of the ideal society, making much use of the analogy of a dance in which individuals are free to move within an overall pattern of movement. The correct individual actions enhance the dance as a whole and vice versa. They hint that a harmonious and fulfilling society fitting the dance analogy may emerge naturally as people come to appreciate the truth of the quantum view of mentality. Rosy pictures are always welcome in a drab world, but a certain amount of scepticism is in order about the likelihood of happy endings if mentality operates along the lines that they favour.

Awareness, they say, is a manifestation of one of a range of possibilities, which one being determined in part by the type of 'measurement' precipitating manifestation. Further, it is subject to non-local correlations between people who are or have been associates. What might one envisage, abandoning rose-coloured spectacles, to be likely results of these two postulates? The short answer is that this looks like a system that will produce positive social feedback, and positive feedback normally leads to runaway outcomes. Much depends on what 'measurement' and 'correlation' might imply in this context. As these terms are used by Zohar and Marshall, they certainly imply reciprocal relationships with overt behaviour:

> If we focus on one quantum entity, we force it into an extreme 'individualist' state . . . If we focus on the group characteristics, we force the entity into an extreme 'collectivist' state where relationship is all and individuality is lost.
>
> (Zohar and Marshall, 1993: 95–6)

> In fact, if we are quantum twins, every time that I am seen to raise my right arm, my twin raises her left one . . . . Each of us chooses freely which arm to raise in the dance. And yet our behaviour is linked as though we are standing in the same room and there are springs connecting our arms.
>
> Zohar and Marshall, 1993: 36)

We are asked to picture, then, social groups in which the mental states of individuals will be correlated not only as a consequence of nature, nurture and education but also through non-local links. Then the 'measurements' made by individuals on each other within these groups will put further constraints on the mental states that can be manifest. No wonder weird sects can mushroom overnight and sinister movements such as Fascism can overthrow the most rational of souls. The terrible thing about this picture is not that it seems wrong but that it fits the facts all too well. No wonder, too, that those who wish to change a society must often first withdraw from it (see, for example, Lehane, 1994, for an interesting account of early Celtic Christianity in which not only was the church itself cut off from the mainstream, but many of its participants isolated themselves for long periods).

All this could be yet another basis for thinking that awareness should have been eliminated by evolution, this time at a stage when animals developed flexible societies. What we have pictured might be all right for coral colonies or shoals of fish, but surely ought to be disadvantageous to creatures like ourselves. Societies that become too way out or too rigid quickly become non-viable; but are there any advantages to be uncovered in the implications of the PM view?

There are two loopholes. The first is that awareness has an inbuilt tendency to realism at the individual level, and this should, to a limited extent translate to its social consequences. There will be a tendency for social consensus to be realistic more often than not. Second, the quantum mechanisms seem to provide a means for achieving rapid consensus throughout a collection of associated individuals. Either of these considerations separately would have adaptive value and the effect of taking them both together would be more than additive. It may well be that short-term gains from this outweigh the long-term disadvantages of rigidity, at least for biological survival, though history would suggest that it may be a different matter as far as the fate of political units and civilisations is concerned.

The completely new factor is that the technological base of our present civilisation is such that collapse could imperil biological survival of the race. It could yet turn out that cultivating awareness was an evolutionary dead end. We clearly need to keep our society as pluralistic as possible, albeit at the risk of multiplying tribal conflicts, so as to preserve nuclei of difference to be drawn on in case of social need. The convergence of abstruse theory and an author's political prejudices no doubt usually gives him a nice warm feeling – and bores readers dreadfully – so it's best to leave this topic now!

WHAT DOES THE BRAIN DO FOR AWARENESS?

Another nonsense question, many would say, but one that is in fact meaningful on a PM perspective with its covert dualism. Proto-awareness, on this view, was around for a long time before brains, at least as a biological potentiality, and maybe even as something that was occasionally realised in coherence effects between large numbers of primitive organisms. For philosophers with a Platonic bent, of course, there is a sense in which awareness must be considered more real than the brains that harbour it. It is consciousness, not brain, that can participate in the world of pure forms and archetypes. Further, it is legitimate to talk about awareness in the singular and brains in the plural since the separate awarenesses of separate brains are interlinked in groupings at all sorts of levels from families through nations to, presumably, the biosphere as a whole. The situation is thus analogous to that found in quantum physics where, for most practical purposes, there is no point in thinking about the wave functions of anything other than single particles but there are some very profound contexts (see Chapter 3) in which one must take account of the wave function of the entire universe.

Clearly, what brains do is to vastly increase the range of shapes that awareness can take. They not only enable it to reflect ever more accurately physical features of the world from a huge number of different angles, they also introduce the elaborate topologies associated with emotional and cognitive sentience. Could all this complexity have potential value to counterbalance the admission of pain into the world? At first sight it would seem not, since awareness is a fleeting series of ghostly entities more insubstantial than autumn leaves blown on the wind.

On second thoughts, however, there is room for doubt. The past is certainly less unreal than is commonly assumed; there would appear to be 'non-temporal' links between past and present similar to the spatially non-local ones that have played so large a part in this book. Indeed, it is correct to define the present as that section of the past/present which divides us from the future. This is in fact tautologous, but the form of words perhaps serves to make the point. The future itself may have some sort of quasi-reality, but cannot be conceived as a continuum with the past/present because wave function collapse occurs at random. These are profound mysteries, but they allow the possibility that the shapes of awareness build structures over time which are as 'solid' as anything else in the universe and have the potential for embellishing its complexity and beauty.

There is, of course, no direct evidence to support this point of view, but there's one pointer worth a mention. Society gives high rewards and considerable resources to a number of groups who have no obvious value or use. Professional sportsmen, artists and historians or archaeologists are obvious examples. Sportsmen are often thought of as surrogate warriors; gladiators with a tincture of the ritual sacrifice as exemplified by Cretan bull dancers or Central American ball players (among whom the captain of the winning team had his heart removed and offered to the Gods). Certainly, they are sometimes crucified by the gutter press and *Gladiators* is a very popular TV programme, but these are probably not their most important roles nowadays. In effect, they show us what our bodies are capable of, or could do if only we were a bit better. One suspects that this is their most important function, in which case they do for the body precisely what we have already proposed that artists do for awareness. They provide us with a mirror and/or an ideal for ourselves. Maybe it is as providers of images in which we can see ourselves (or our better selves) that both sportsmen and artists are so highly valued.

Historians are to some extent sought after as tellers of strange tales of times remote and places far, but on the whole they are not so good at this as fantasy writers. Some (e.g. Spengler, Toynbee) claim to discern patterns in historical events of use for predicting the future and are avidly read in an upmarket version of the spirit that leads people to Nostrodamus or an astrology column in the paper. The most respected of all, however, (e.g. Trevelyan or Taylor in this country, Braudel in France) simply try to 'tell it as it was' and some among them have emphasised that the main lesson of history is that there is no lesson of history – there are no patterns to be discerned of use for predicting the future. Why should these people be valued? Intellectual curiosity no doubt plays a large part, but there are many things which might attract equal curiosity while lacking the social standing of historical studies. It is just possible that historians should be thought of as the artists who depict the structures erected by awareness over time, and an intuition that this is so has been responsible for the apparently anomalous regard in which they are held.

CONCLUSIONS

Probably enough has been said to indicate that the PM paradigm has biological plausibility and can provide insights into a range of social and related phenomena. One could continue along this line at inordinate length, eventually encroaching on theological realms, but to do so would in a sense be only to build castles in the air, at least until such time as we have more conclusive evidence that PM ideas are nearer to the truth than HE ones. What I hope to have indicated is that, if the PM paradigm should turn out to be securely founded, the castles would prove spacious, elegant and generally well worth building from the points of view of a wide range of people and their special interests.

There may be value in describing the more detailed implications of our paradigm for one specific field. As my own special interest is medicine in general and psychiatry in particular, the next Chapter will be occupied with looking at what the castles might be like that relate to this field, and indeed with the question of whether a detailed look will also provide evidence reflecting on the validity of the paradigm itself.

REFERENCES

Dawkins, M.S. (1993) *Through Our Eyes Only? The Search for Animal Consciousness*, W.H. Freeman: Oxford.

Humphrey, N. (1986) *The Inner Eye*, Faber: London.

Humphrey, N. (1992) *A History of the Mind*, Chatto & Windus: London.

Hundert, E.M. (1987) 'Can Neuroscience Contribute to Philosophy?', in *Mindwaves*, C. Blakemore and S. Greenfield (eds), Basil Blackwell: Oxford.

Jaynes, J. (1990) *The Origin of Consciousness in the Breakdown of the Bicameral Mind*, Houghton Mifflin: Boston.

Lehane, B. (1994) *Early Celtic Christianity*, Constable: London.

Newman, D.J. (1994) 'The Origin of Consciousness in the Relativistic Brain', (paper to be published).

Penrose, R. (1994) *Shadows of the Mind*, Oxford University Press.

van der Post, L. (1962) *The Soul of the White Ant*, Penguin Books: Harmondsworth.

Zohar, D. and Marshall, I. (1993) *The Quantum Society*, Bloomsbury: London.

8 Medicine and the PM paradigm

Right at the beginning of this book, the 'obvious' statement was made that you can't have awareness without a brain to have it in. This was a bit rash and has now to be qualified a good deal in the light of all that has been discussed. It appears that you probably can't have awareness without an energy-using cellular mechanism to originate it, and you can't have any very complex or sophisticated awareness without a brain to modulate it. We have not discovered anything to prevent us from supposing that cells other than those in the brain might sometimes directly participate in forming the structures which comprise awareness. Whether this is a real possibility would depend on (unknown) details of the basis of the Bose condensation. But maybe, when a gymnast, for instance, performs one of her amazing feats, consciousness really does centre in her muscles. Perhaps those odd visceral sensations that we all get from time to time are at least partly derived from one's stomach or wherever and are not wholly a cerebral reaction to information coming over autonomic nervous pathways – though central systems must also be involved or the sensations could not be remembered or reported.

As it turns out, these ideas could allow revival of a rather subtle version of the old (and discredited) James–Lange theory which regarded emotions as resulting from physical responses to cerebral events. The sensation of fear, for instance, was said to be the result of adrenaline release making your heart pound, your face blanch, etc. Although it is now known that emotions can be felt without any overt somatic change, there's nothing to prevent us from supposing that under normal, as opposed to experimental, conditions bodily happenings may sometimes directly add their quota to a quale. There's perhaps no very strong incentive for wanting to revive such an antique idea, except that it has always had a strong appeal because it has felt right to many among generations of psychologists, even though latterly thought false at an intellectual level. Also, it sets the scene for the introduction of our first medical topic. This is because, as has already been argued, awareness in the form of Bose condensation can affect the function of neurones; if it sometimes involves other cells as well, there is no reason why it should not affect them too – for good or ill. So it's possible to suppose that direct, two-way interactions between mind and body may occur in addition to the rather indirect chains of causation that are more commonly envisaged. Ho (1994) has in fact argued at some length that a great many biological processes, including muscle contraction, rely on long-range quantum coherence effects of a similar type to those producing consciousness on the PM view. The probability that 'muscle fields', among others, would sometimes get entangled with 'awareness fields' is high if she (Ho) is right.

PSYCHOSOMATIC MEDICINE

This is sometimes referred to instead as 'holistic' medicine, a term which has been largely appropriated nowadays by alternative practitioners to whom it seems to mean a range of different things. To some it appears to imply that, if you are at one with nature by only eating natural things (they exclude botulinus toxin, for instance, from the list of these), then you will be happy and healthy in body and mind for evermore; others have ideas about how body and soul must be in harmony and propound a variety of prescriptions for achieving this, often derived from Asian practices or philosophies.

As recently as 30 years ago, however, the whole subject was of major interest to mainstream medicine and attracted much research. Selye (1950) had published his theory that all disease is a manifestation of what he termed the 'general adaptational syndrome' – a standard response to stress of all types. Dunbar (1954) had written her monumental review of research in the field since 1910, which included over 5000 references. Hinckle and Wolff's very influential paper appeared in 1957. This gave the results of a huge and meticulously conducted study showing that people's illnesses (of all types both mental and physical) tended to occur in clusters at times in their lives when they were having to cope with social upheavals. As late as 1968, Leigh, a pillar of the medical establishment at the time, could write a weighty article in praise of the holistic approach to medicine.

This whole field is now of only the most peripheral interest to the average doctor, partly because research into it was prone to circularity and to giving ambiguous outcomes, though no worse in this respect than other areas of enquiry (the relation between nutrition and heart disease, for instance) that attract major continuing interest. The main reason is philosophic; a holistic approach simply came to appear silly and unproductive compared to looking for specific cures for specific diseases. At about the time that Hinckle and Wolff were doing their research, whole hospitals were being closed down as a consequence of the discovery of specific, effective drug treatments for tuberculosis (TB). All the research that had been done on social antecedents and personality correlates of TB, which was voluminous and now entirely forgotten, began to seem a waste of time and this attitude carried over to other fields. The final nail in the coffin of holism's popularity probably came from the discovery of diuretics. Before these came into general use, around 1960, every medical ward had had its colony of patients with dropsy. These unfortunates were in a terrible predicament with hugely swollen legs, usually due to chronic heart disease, that had to be daily tapped for fluid rather as a rubber tree is tapped. They are hardly ever to be met now that the right drugs are available. Some disenchantment with the search for specific cures was beginning to appear by the 1980s, which probably led to the upsurge in 'alternative' holistic treatments at that time and might also have resulted in renewed medical interest had it not been for the allure and early achievement of developments in molecular biology which have swept all before them.

This is not to say that the psychosomatic approach has entirely died. It has not. The *Journal of Psychosomatic Research* is still going strong. Much 1960s-like work is still carried out; for example, that of Cooper and Faragher (1993) who showed that certain types of coping strategy and personality make people more liable to develop breast cancer following untoward and unpleasant stress. What has happened, though, is that the whole approach has been sidelined in the minds of most doctors.

It's not new for the psychosomatic approach to disease to undergo violent swings in popularity. For instance Morgagni (1761) was proposing a sophisticated psychosomatic hypothesis when he wrote (about gallstones):

> Yet the middle age, although it is an active season of life, has not the juices to be compared with the flourishing prime of our age, for which reason it happens that this time of life cannot equally withstand the injuries of intemperance and of the passions.

Just over a hundred years later Da Costa (1871) wrote about his syndrome, also called 'effort syndrome', in quite a different spirit. This condition prevented recruits for the Spanish-American war, and subsequently the First World War, from walking more than a few steps without severe fatigue. Da Costa never considered the possibility that it might be due to anything other than a specific, if subtle, cardiac lesion!

The lesson to be derived from all this is that there are two valid ways of looking at disease which are to some extent mutually exclusive and so tend to see-saw in popularity. One approach considers psychic and somatic factors to be closely interwoven or inseparable in the causation of illness, and usually brings in social circumstances too. The other sees only a range of discrete conditions with precisely identifiable (in principle) causes.

Both of these approaches fit in all right with the HE paradigm, in which there is no distinction between mental and brain events: the brain is part of the soma, so psyche and soma are inseparable. Malfunctions in such a system could have general origins, in stress reactions, for example, as well as specific causes of various types. It is all rather bland and provides no basis for the tension that has persisted for so long between the two different outlooks on how illness should be regarded.

PM ideas are rather different in this respect as well as in so many others. There is potentially a difference between psychic and somatic disorders because of the limited dualism entailed by PM theories. We shall look in more detail later on at which conditions, if any, might be thought primarily psychic. These ideas also involve a type of holism, beyond the scope of the HE paradigm, deriving from non-local links that join people with each other and with their environments. The medical consequences of this, too, merit further exploration in due course. Perhaps it is the inherent tension between dualistic and holistic consequences of the PM paradigm that has surfaced in a distorted form in debates over psychosomatic medicine and caused the violent shifts in outlook that have been described. Similar switches of opinion occurred between wave and particle theories of light before quantum theory was developed, probably for equivalent reasons.

To elaborate on this point, Roessler and Greenfield (1961), in the most recent heyday of psychosomatic medicine, could write that the appearance of dualism in psychosomatic studies is 'more a function of experimental bias and perspective than a reflection of actual dichotomous events'. This is a statement that must appear just plain silly nowadays to any doctor willing to think about it. Innumerable studies have shown that psychic and somatic changes, though some-times associated in one way or another, are more often unrelated. A relevant example (Nunn, 1974) followed the progression of physical and mental symptoms, plus social circumstances, in a group of ill old people. Physical and 'organic' mental symptoms (such as memory loss and cognitive impairment) did indeed seem closely bound up with one another, but symptoms of emotional disturbance followed an almost entirely independent course apart from a few common-sense associations (e.g. having severe heart disease can make you anxious; being immobile because of arthritis makes it difficult to get over any depression).

A claim could of course be made that any appearance of dualism is illusory because it's a consequence of emotional disturbances, say, being caused by dysfunction of a different part of the soma from that resulting in memory loss or indigestion. What is really going on can be described by the ugly term 'somatic multi-axialism' which sometimes gives rise to the appearance of dualism. This is not, however, what Roessler and Greenfield wanted to imply; they envisaged some profound unity, of psyche with soma and environment, underlying all appearances of separate entities. This intuition is almost without meaning in most medical circles at present but is nevertheless one that keeps coming back. If orthodox medicine won't entertain it, then alternative practitioners flourish. It may well reflect some aspect of reality.

In brief, both holism and a degree of dualism may be valid concepts in relation to psychic and somatic aspects of medicine. The situation is reminiscent of conflicts of evidence and opinion about the wave or particle theories of light which occurred before quantum theory was developed basically because, we are claiming here, both approaches are true. Both are aspects of a quantum reality. It's not just a matter of semantic problems or difficulty in disentangling specific from general causes of disease.

ARE THERE ANY PSYCHIC ILLNESSES?

To the HE enthusiast, the answer has to be 'Not really'. Mind words such as 'psyche' are only partially meaningful in relation to behaviours, including illness behaviours; they are ersatz substitutes for the correct brain (i.e somatic) words that we would use about the immediate antecedents of mental illness if only we were not so ignorant. The phrase 'psychosomatic medicine' is itself indicative of a profound conceptual error in medical philosophy since the adjective should be 'somatosomatic' which is tautologous unless qualified by making the division between the two 'somas' refer to, say, the blood-brain barrier.

On PM ideas psychic diseases can be defined as disorders of Bose condensates forming the basis of awareness, which are not due to primary abnormality of the underlying, classical, neural machinery. This is not the place to pursue any deep enquiry into the meaning of the terms 'illness', 'disease' or 'disorder'. They will be regarded simply as implying abnormalities of function sufficient to cause distress to their possessor and/or his or her close associates. How might primary disorders of the Bose condensates show themselves?

It's tempting to follow up the hint offered by Robbie Burns:

> Human bodies are such fools,
> For all their colleges and schools,
> That when no real ills perplex them,
> They make enough themselves to vex them.

Maybe one should look for primarily psychic diseases among the fashionable ills that come and go almost as fast as hemlines rise and fall. However, one has to tread warily, as the example of eating disorders shows. These (anorexia, bulimia) are often regarded as quintessentially psychic illnesses, becoming ever more prevalent as magazine and newspaper articles spread their fame, and clearly based either on a revulsion from the consumerist culture which has been rammed down sufferers' throats or, more likely, on the ill effects of trying to make females' shape conform to male ideals which have become increasingly unnatural since the days of Reubens.

Despite this apparently convincing case, a proportion of those with the most experience of treating eating disorders have always suspected that they may be based on primary abnormalities of brain appetite-regulating centres. The current favourite (Treasure and Campbell, 1994) is that anorexia may be due to overactive serotonin pathways in the hypothalamus and related areas. Moreover, eating disorders have always been around. Four of the terms currently used to describe them have been applied in the same way to delineate similar cases from the fourteenth century onwards (Parry-Jones, 1991).

Actually, it's an implication of the PM paradigm that two different types of primarily psychic illness should exist; the first based on abnormalities unique to an individual of his/her Bose condensates and the second on abnormalities in a population due to non-local links between people's condensates. The latter type, in particular, may seize upon and amplify somatic predispositions existing in the population as grist to its mill. These predispositions, before 'psychic' amplification, will not amount to somatic illnesses in most individuals but may do so in a few. It is thus to be expected that 'psychic' factors will sometimes serve as transmission mechanisms for what would otherwise be rare somatic diseases, so causing puzzles for epidemiologists and those concerned with aetiology. Although this proposal may provide one way of accounting for some of the conceptual problems centring around eating disorders and the like, it has not really helped to disentangle primary psychic illness from somatic illness; indeed it's added yet another source of entanglement!

When looking for possible examples of sporadic primary psychic illness occurring in individuals there are three fairly obvious candidates for consideration. First, psychogenic pain, which can be of crippling severity. Trethowan (1988) described a case of a lady whose problems were 'pain and trouble with her husband'. She could describe the pain in terms of intensity but not quality. She used expressions like 'a terrific pain – very bad; definitely a bad pain; a pain that really hurts; a sore pain'. She was evidently recounting an experience that was real to her but lacked some of the qualities of organic pain, perhaps because there was no input to the relevant primary pain maps. Trethowan concluded about her:

> In essence there seems little doubt that her symptoms were the means by which she could cope with her marital difficulties. Her pain, in effect, absolved her from having to do anything about her marriage, for, underneath it all, she seemed to be aware that she was emotionally dependent on her husband and that however much she disliked him she could not do without him

The PM account of her condition is a bit different but quite simple; for her, the mental representations of her marital circumstances had a similar shape to the representations that she recalled of organic pains. It would be possible to arrive at related conclusions of either sort via an HE route, but the road would be long and circuitous.

The next candidate is especially interesting in that sufferers from it directly say that there is something wrong with their awareness. The depersonalisation/derealisation syndrome has been defined in one recent textbook (Hughes, 1991) as 'a sensation of dream-like unreality of the self/outside world', but actually is more complex and sometimes more dramatic than this implies. Part or the whole of the body can appear to change in size or some other subjective quality; people can be distressed by a feeling that they can't feel anything, 'as if I'd turned into a robot'; they can think themselves cut off from the whole outside world as if behind a sheet of glass. Despite protestations that there is something drastically wrong with themselves or their experience, they appear from an outsider's point of view to be functioning entirely normally. They don't appear in the least dreamy or otherwise impaired. Even people who say that they feel as if they cannot feel or remember anything answer memory tests correctly and have normal emotional responsiveness. The syndrome is often secondary to another psychiatric condition (e.g. schizophrenia, depression, anxiety state), and is occasionally a consequence of temporal lobe epilepsy, but can happen on its own. When secondary it will usually clear up along with the underlying disorder but, when primary, there is no known treatment and it can persist for years. Maybe it's a disorder of Bose condensates that is not always secondary to dysfunction of classical brain systems. It could prove a good starting point for research on awareness.

The final candidate is a type of delayed post-traumatic stress syndrome. Most psychiatrists have had experience of a few cases, but it is difficult to convey an impression of their all-consuming quality and intensity to those who have never seen one. One that I met was a middle-aged lady who had lived an entirely normal and successful adult life. Then, for no obvious reason, she had disturbing dreams for a few nights after which she started to fluctuate during the daytime in and out of a strange state in which she was hallucinated and behaving like a 5-year-old. This state became continuous for several days during which she hardly slept at all. As it became continuous she started to recount in an entirely childish way what was, from her point of view, actually happening to her at the time, although the events themselves had occurred nearly fifty years previously. While her father was away at the war, an elderly neighbour had taken to enticing her into his coal-shed and sexually abusing her with the usual threats about what would happen if she told anyone. In fact she did not tell anyone, not so much through fear as because she knew how her mother was finding it hard to cope, and she did not want to add to mother's burdens. The condition remitted as it had come on – her adult self started to reappear at intervals, then there were only troubled dreams and within about three weeks she was fully back to her normal self. The only 'treatment' was letting her talk (to her husband and myself); she was given no drugs or the like. There are accounts of such phenomena in terms of repressed memories, repressed complexes, etc. It's a lot simpler to think that this lady was reliving the trauma that she had been through in some sort of real and direct manner. But it is hard to envisage how classical neural systems could achieve the necessary immediacy after so long; the PM account, which allows the possibility of non-temporal links between past events and present experience, is perhaps less difficult to believe – at least for people who have witnessed the extraordinary intensity and immediacy involved in such occurrences.

It might be thought odd to omit cases of personality disorder from a list of possible primary psychic dysfunctions. The problem with them is that their status is so uncertain. Some are clearly based on inherited deviations from the norm of brain architecture or function, others on trauma or infections interfering with brain development, yet others on adverse factors in the social environment. There may indeed be some which are based on a consistent misuse of 'free will' by a semi-independent psyche. However, speculation about this is fairly pointless in the absence of much knowledge about the more basic types of personality disorder. Moreover, if any such conditions occur, they might be better thought of as habitual vices than as medical quasi-illnesses.

It's worth going into a bit more detail about the possible shared or epidemic forms of psychic illness. Some are very ephemeral and never really get a hold. Readers will probably recall the quite frequent newspaper articles, around ten years ago, concerning people suffering total allergy to the twentieth century who would collapse if they emerged from sterile rooms with a filtered air supply and had to be taken on special flights for esoteric treatments in America. Although some of the original cases still retain their symptoms, they seem to be a dying breed as new recruits are now extremely rare.

Chronic fatigue syndromes are more widespread and persistent. They share a lot of the general characteristics of eating disorders, though the actual symptoms are quite different from those of eating disorder. Fatigue itself is a very poorly understood symptom from the physiological point of view but certainly has a large subjective (i.e. mental) component. People have always been liable to suffer excessive fatiguability without any obvious organic disease to account for it. Da Costa's syndrome is an example. At one time they were often given the diagnosis of 'neurasthenia'. Wessely (1990) rather cynically pointed out that:

> Neurasthenia retained its popularity as a diagnosis for as long as it was viewed as a non-psychiatric, neurological illness caused by environmental factors which affected successful people and for which the cure was rest.

This condition is now reincarnated as ME (Myalgic encephalomyelitis). A few sufferers may have some obscure virus affecting their mitochondria (the cellular organs which produce energy) or whatever, but there's a lot of research to indicate that the symptoms of most patients are partly or wholly of mental origin. A recent study (Wood *et al.*, 1994), for example, compared ME sufferers, psychiatric out-patients and muscular dystrophy patients. They were asked to rate their physical and mental symptoms before and after a mildly stressful task (twenty minutes of solving anagrams). The ME sufferers had the greatest increase in symptoms of both types; the muscular dystrophy sufferers, who were certainly prone to primary muscular fatigue, experienced *the least* increase in symptoms. The researchers thought that their findings might be due to an abnormality of attention resulting in ME patients noticing symptoms more than the other groups. There is no simple 'organic' hypothesis that can account for their getting more physical as well as mental symptoms than people known to have muscular fatiguability of physical origin after purely mental stress.

Many ME victims are like the patient who could not walk for more than a few yards or tidy her room without suffering immediate exhaustion and a need to do nothing whatsoever for a day or two after. She would be ferried to out-patients by concerned friends where she would discuss her symptoms at inordinate length and with such vivacity and force that one felt quite exhausted oneself at being on the receiving end of all the energy she put into it! Unfortunates like her are surely suffering some disorder of awareness that is so persistent over time and so widely shared that it has an archetypal quality.

It's not at all clear how many diseases might be like ME in having a large primary psychic component. Illnesses of this type tend to fluctuate widely in popularity and prevalence from time to time for unknown reasons. Epidemiologists and critics of Western medicine (such as Ivan Illich, the author of *Medical Nemesis*) point out that the prevalence of major diseases has often started to decline a decade or more *before* the introduction of effective new treatments for them. This was true of tuberculosis, peptic ulcer (long thought to be a psychosomatic condition, though now attributed by some to a specific bacterial infection) and heart disease if one regards coronary bypass surgery and other new treatments as particularly effective (still a matter for debate). It's a phenomenon which could be due solely to specific factors such as hygiene improvements, changes of diet, etc., but there's room to wonder whether it may not also have a 'psychic' component; however, the evidence is not sufficiently good to let one do more than wonder.

The status of most psychiatric illnesses is equally uncertain. Some (e.g. schizophrenia, obsessive-compulsive disorder, many depressions) are likely to be mainly somatic in that they are probably entirely due to disorders of classical neuronal systems. The so-called culture-bound syndromes such as Koro (an acute fear that one's penis may be about to shrink into one's abdomen with fatal consequences) seem good candidates for being ME-like. Agoraphobia should perhaps be included among these since it probably reached an apogee in popularity twenty or thirty years ago, and new cases are less common than they were. One cannot be at all sure about there being a primary psychic component in the causation of these illnesses, though, because they can all be regarded as manifestations of anxiety/depressive disorder which could be entirely somatic. Psychic factors may modify presentation without actually causing illness. If this were the case one would expect an increase in the incidence of generalised panic disorder, for example, to precisely balance a decline in that of agoraphobia, other things being equal. The epidemiological evidence is not good enough to tell whether or not this is what happens, at least partly because other things never are quite equal and it's very difficult to partial out their effects on the results obtained from studies.

All things considered, it appears likely that primary psychic disorder peculiar to an individual is quite rare and often caused by psychic trauma of one sort or another. The most widespread and important psychic disorders are those shared with many other people that may have a basis in somatic predisposition or susceptibility which does not by itself amount to illness. They behave a bit like infectious diseases and are based on archetype-like mental entities.

ARCHETYPES

Jung himself, who first pinpointed the important role of archetypes in the psyche, originally considered them inborn though his later views were more variable. The following quotation, written in 1939, indicates clearly what he was thinking then:

> But we soon come up against the fact that, in its basic structure, the human psyche is as little personalistic as the body. It is far rather something inherited and universal. The logic of the intellect, the *raison du coeur*, the emotions, the instincts, the basic images and forms of imagination, have in a way more resemblance to Kant's table of *a priori* categories or to Plato's *eida* than to the scurrilities, circumstantialities, whims and tricks of our personal minds.

Most people nowadays would agree that instincts, say, and some of the 'logic of the intellect' (e.g. the deep structure of grammar) have a genetic basis, but we would not be so sure about the 'basic images and forms of imagination'. As has already been pointed out (Chapter 7), the PM view can and has been interpreted in a manner that adds force and substance to what is almost a truism; namely that groupings of people tend to share awarenesses that may have a pervasive influence on the content of each individual mind. These shared images have the characteristics which Jung envisaged for his archetypes but are more various, flexible and readily engendered than he may have considered.

At the most permanent level there are racial awarenesses of, say, the Bountiful Mother or the Wise Old Man. The myths of any particular civilisation also contain figures, such as that of Orpheus, that are not necessarily shared with other cultures. It's amusing to look for national archetypes, too. An obvious British one is the Horatio Nelson – the game, but maimed little man who nevertheless gets the women and one up on the opposition. His latest, though incomplete, incarnation was in 'Eddie the Eagle' who failed so conspicuously to do well in the Winter Olympic ski jumping, but nevertheless got all the publicity. He shows subtle differences from related figures in other nations (e.g. Woody Allen in America or the Good Soldier Schweik in the former Czechoslovakia; he's less intellectual than the first and more of an extrovert than the second, among other distinguishing features). These archetypes, or stereotypes if you prefer, go all the way down through quite small organisations, where they are often referred to under the categories of 'ethos' or 'morale', to individual family units. The image of the kindly but tight-fisted Yorkshireman really does bias the content of the consciousness of many people from Leeds. Traditions of public service or whatever in a family can shape the course of whole lives.

Unhappily, these quasi-entities are not always benign. The most devastating psychic diseases have their origin in malignant archetypes, though they are generally classified as illnesses only if the relevant archetype is of the sort hinted at by Wessely (i.e. the Good Person Cast Down in Their Prime by Disease Unknown to Medical Science). The archetypes in question may be inherently malignant, for instance, the Hag That Devours Children and Men who has recently awoken in people's imaginations, along with some old cronies such as the Warlock, in scares over satanic abuse, or they may come to life in contexts in which they do harm. O'Donnell (1994) has written amusingly about the Wise Friend:

> when a friend who had suffered an emotional trauma declined an offer of help from a nurse-counsellor, the nurse-counsellor turned quite nasty. Her manner. . . which had previously been unctuously concerned, became harsh and vindictive. . . This ill-defined activity called counselling is certainly in fashion. Victims, even witnesses of accidents and other tragedies are assumed to be in need of it as. . . is anyone who suffers a condition for which medicine cannot provide a quick therapeutic fix. . . Too many people who call themselves

'professional counsellors' act as though the title implies that they have access to wisdom denied to the rest of us and the authority to tell us what is good for us.

The point is not that people in distress don't need friendship and sensible advice but that the counsellors themselves sometimes act as if they had been taken over by an entity which distorts their own personalities and harms those they would have wished to help. Since it is acceptable to talk about 'iatrogenic' (i.e. doctor-induced) diseases, it should also be all right to refer to this sort of process as a disease.

The most devastating conditions of all, of course, occur when the Hero or the Messiah comes to life in a stressed society that fails to contain him. Napoleon and Hitler were of this ilk. Having been given life by their societies, they can hardly be blamed as individuals for living the part to its end in ruin. They were in the same situation as a carrier of plague – they could not have known for sure what they were incubating until it was too late. Nor could anyone else have been sure in advance that their societies lacked the necessary 'antibodies' to neutralise them or confine them to some area in which they could have been useful.

CURES FOR THE PSYCHE?

These have of course always been around, but our paradigm points to new avenues for exploration and throws fresh light on some old ones. A completely new possibility, that might lead to symptomatic treatment for a proportion of both primary and secondary disorders of awareness, would involve the use of microwaves. Awareness requires energy and energy use is decreased in particular brain areas in many psychiatric illnesses (see Chapter 1). Decreased use is likely to be most often due to abnormalities of classical neuronal function, though conceivably it might sometimes be due to primary psychic disorder. However, the energy produced by the classical systems provides the source for that used in the quantum systems, so the two are related. Classical systems metabolise chemicals to create electrochemical events. In the Frohlich/ Hameroff version, consequences of some of the electrical events provide the basis for condensates; however, they depend on only a proportion of the total energy produced – that which powers microwave frequency vibrations in dipoles of one sort or another. If microwave energy is sometimes deficient in a particular area, due to illness from whatever cause, there is no reason in principle why one should not supply it directly by beaming waves of the right frequency to the affected brain area.

Of course, one would have to know what frequency to use and precisely where it should be directed in order to do any good. It would also be important not to supply so much energy as to actually cook the brain! Further, the proposal would only work if awareness is based on condensates of phonons, not if it is based on Goldstone bosons or other exotic particles. All the same, it is intriguing to think that someone with severe depression, say, might be made to feel entirely well by beaming microwaves at his left frontal lobe. The technique might eventually come to be used as a diagnostic test as well as a sort of 'psychic aspirin' particularly as people with areas of *excess* energy use would either not be helped or perhaps made to feel worse. Once the basic groundwork had been done, it would presumably be quicker and cheaper for some purposes than expensive tests like PET or fast MRI.

There's also an intriguing possibility of a more direct route towards testing for abnormalities of awareness; that is to directly measure microwaves radiated by different areas of the brain. The main problem with this approach would be that such waves are expected to have a very low field strength of the order of only one five-thousandth of a volt per metre (Tourenne, 1985). It would need a major effort to come up with apparatus capable of detecting them.

To revert to less futuristic considerations, it has to be remembered that people have almost always thought that they might have a 'psychic' side to their natures and have had methods for trying to put right some of the ills attributed to this aspect of themselves. Perhaps their treatments were sometimes effective. A problem is that cures for the psyche have tended to get muddled up with punishments for crime and methods of promoting religious conformity and belief, to such an extent that it's often not clear what the primary aim of a given method might be.

The methods of witch doctors, however, provide an example of relatively uncontaminated attempts to cure. The underlying belief is that many ills are due to malevolent spells or wishes, or sometimes to witting or unwitting infringement of taboos. In most cultures where this belief system is prevalent witch-doctors may be willing to inflict harm as well as relieve it, though in Africa at least they tend to specialise; you go to a 'bad' witch doctor if you want a curse put on a rival or to a 'good' one if you have symptoms that suggest having been cursed and you want relief. It is known which doctor to go to for which purpose!

Sargant (1957) has described a method of cure that is seen in a wide range of cultures. He also thought that it is often effective, though there are of course no double-blind controlled trials of it in the literature. He was interested in religious and political conversions, techniques of brainwashing, as well as cures. He speculated that what happens in these circumstances has much in common with the emotional changes and switches of behaviour that Pavlov observed in dogs under stress. When a dog enters a state of what Pavlov termed 'transmarginal inhibition' it becomes abnormally susceptible to environmental influences as if lightly hypnotised; as it progresses to the phase of 'protective inhibition', previous behaviour patterns tend to reverse so that the dog shows hatred for what it had earlier loved and vice versa. These ideas have recently been reassessed by Birtchnell (1994) who thinks that they have validity and wonders why they have been so neglected for so long.

A typical curative technique of witch-doctors is to induce a state in their patients certainly analogous to, and perhaps identical with, 'transmarginal inhibition' by means of a long, sometimes all night, session of rhythmic drumming, dancing and clapping. Then at what he judges to be the right moment, the doctor will make a 'diagnosis', saying that he has identified the source of the spell, for instance, quickly followed by the 'cure'. The latter may simply be to state that the spell is now removed or may be something more elaborate as in the case of the Far Eastern healers who appear to extract a rotten organ (the alleged source of the problem) from their patients by sleight of hand. It's usually very much a group activity in which relatives and the whole village join. This probably speeds the process. When carried out in isolation there generally has to be a long preparatory phase, often involving fasting or other privation. Sargant drew detailed analogies between this process and that of psychoanalysis, though in his opinion psychoanalysis is an activity that tends more to the brainwashing end of the spectrum and is a long way from being straightforwardly curative.

In summary, the typical traditional 'psychic' cure involves getting the patient into an abnormal mental state in which he is unusually suggestible and unusually likely to reverse previous beliefs and behaviours. This can be achieved most quickly in a group setting; either privation or a great deal of time are needed to get comparable results in isolation. Then at the crucial moment a new, hopefully curative, belief is suggested to the patient.

Even though psychoanalysis itself is now almost defunct, there is much in the traditional technique that is used by contemporary psychotherapies. To be precise, two of the main features are consciously used nowadays while the third and probably the most important, that of inducing a state of transmarginal inhibition, is quite neglected by most psychotherapists despite the fact that it has remained popular, for very different purposes, with interrogators, torturers, religious fundamentalists and their ilk.

The powerful effect of groups has been widely recognised ever since the Second World War when group therapy was found to be an effective means of treating neuroses due to trauma. For instance Munich (1993) comments in a standard textbook on group psychotherapy: 'That individual dynamic (i.e. the individual person's way of looking at things) rapidly develops into a group level phenomenon and becomes a shared experience'.

As far as one-to-one therapy is concerned, a method that has been shown to be more effective than other comparable contemporary treatments for many problems, particularly mild to moderate depression, is cognitive therapy. This consists in essence of getting the patient to clearly state his beliefs on a range of sensitive topics and then to persistently suggest alternatives to those that appear dysfunctional. Examples of dysfunctional beliefs might be: 'I'm always second best', 'I'll always lose if I try to stand up to authority'. Ideas like these tend to lurk in the background of all our lives doing harm, but can be brought into awareness with a little effort and can then be shown up as sometimes untrue. It's a nice, rational treatment that appeals to nice, rational therapists and congenial patients. Although it might be more effective and more widely applicable if techniques of inducing transmarginal inhibition were incorporated, it would also become far murkier and more risky; best, maybe, to let it continue in a pure form.

How can these three components of effective therapy, transmarginal inhibition, group phenomena and belief change, be viewed in terms of our paradigms? One might anticipate that HE ideas will have the advantage in relation to the first which involves brain words, while PM ideas may fit more naturally with the other two as they are usually described in mind words. It's best to take them one by one.

Unfortunately, there are no clear ideas about what is going on in neurological terms when states of abnormal suggestibility are induced. There's probably some relationship between hypnotic states and those described by Pavlov, but this is not of much help as the nature of hypnosis is very obscure. Though Pavlov was using brain words, they can be understood only in terms of mind words when one tries to extend his concepts to cover phenomena in human beings. This may be simply a reflection of our present ignorance. If permanently true, however, it would provide an interesting counter-example to the current mainstream assumption that many mind words will eventually be subsumed in brain ones.

At least for the present, one has to say that the 'will' becomes detached from determining action and belief in these states and its place is taken by external influences of various sorts. Meanwhile, beliefs become labile perhaps because they are no longer reinforced by the person's own mind. This implies a degree of dualism which does not fit comfortably with the HE approach. It's not a strong argument against the HE line because the appearance of dualism may be due to semantic problems rather than anything more fundamental. All the same, it is tempting to think that the varied paraphernalia involved in inducing hypnotic-like states serve the purpose of detaching Bose condensates from such close involvement as normally occurs with the main flow of classical brain activity, and attaching them to externals of one sort or another.

One might even be able to construct a hypnosis machine for carrying out the process more efficiently. This would be an apparatus not unlike the one used in the Southampton experiment (see Chapter 5). It would induce wave function collapse in, say, the occipital cortex by moving a weight in synchrony with the alpha rhythm there and would also show synchronous pictures of something outside the person's everyday experience; a series of those nice computer generated images of ever finer detail in a Mandelbrot set would be a good choice (why, incidentally, are the fractal patterns of a Mandelbrot set perceived as lovely? An ability to answer this question would indicate a true understanding of aesthetics). A machine like this ought to keep anyone's Bose condensates fully occupied. When used in therapy, helpful influences of some sort could be directed at a patient's parallel classical systems while his Bose condensates were engaged elsewhere. At present, of course, this is only a fantasy but something like it could quickly become a reality if PM ideas turn out to be as valid as the indications so far suggest.

The powerful effect of groups is due, in PM terms, to non-local links which can so readily be established between the awarenesses of associates, resulting in the development of what we have described as 'archetypes', thus stretching the usual meaning of the term a bit. Any therapist who finds that the archetype of the Healer has come to life in his group, centred on himself, has a head start. The skill, of course, comes in using archetypes like this constructively; they can very easily run amok and create havoc when either skill or wisdom are lacking. A PM group psychotherapy would use archetypes in a far more conscious way than is usual nowadays. It would need to resurrect many of the ideas of Jungian therapists tempered with a wholly new flexibility in the use of archetypes, plus an irreverence for them that few Jungians manage to achieve.

Perhaps surprisingly HE ideas, too, provide a basis for understanding the effectiveness of groups. The neural representations of role models and the like can be readily pictured as having a powerful modifying influence on all the other reflexive neural activity that is going on, aided no doubt by inbuilt mechanisms for achieving social cohesion that may have evolved over the millennia (mechanisms analogous to the submission postures of dogs and wolves which prevent them from harming one another). It has been known for several decades that the most powerful influence on the outcome of any psychotherapy has something to do with the personality of the therapist. In fact, what the therapist is like is more important to outcome than the type of psychotherapy he uses. This can and has been taken to support claims about the primary importance of suitable role models and similar influences which perhaps sit a little more comfortably with HE ideas than PM ones.

Belief is a very odd thing, particularly when considered in the light of Marcel's (see Chapter 1) conclusions. Even if driven by emotion, it's essentially a cognitive phenomenon. Therefore, one would expect every possible cognitive aspect of whatever a particular belief is concerned with to be available to the brain. Yet one aspect only is often seized upon, sometimes so firmly that even when it is patently false to outsiders a person may be willing to kill or die in defence of its validity. The HE paradigm can deal fairly adequately with delusory beliefs associated with sporadic mental illness. One can always postulate that the illness has knocked off most of a brain's parallel cognitive channels leaving the field to only one contender, or that some neural upset has occurred which allows only one of multiple candidates to ever gain access to a global workspace.

The latter idea (restricted access to a global workspace) might be stretched to account for a dysfunctional belief held by a normal brain; perhaps there was something in their constitution or previous experience which led to the neural embodiment of a particular cognitive angle having an especially good 'fit' with that person's workspace. Epidemic beliefs, such as those associated with fatigue syndromes, might occur when constitution and 'education' had prepared the ground in a sufficient number of global workspaces. Once the idea has been stretched this far, however, various difficulties with it begin to crop up. There is the surprising readiness with which very disparate people can be so quickly subsumed into a group awareness that often takes the form of a shared belief. There is the fact that beliefs often convert, not into agnosticism or a balanced acceptance of all possibilities which is what one might expect to happen in normal brains on the HE paradigm, but into a sometimes opposed alternative. Finally, there is the fact that one might have expected such a faculty to have been eliminated by evolution, or at least rendered extremely rare, since it would appear to incur all the evolutionary penalties that we envisaged for awareness in previous Chapters with none of the advantages that the PM view allows. Each of these objections could be overcome by special pleading of one sort or another, but really the PM view with its shared 'archetypes' offers a much simpler account!

How best to cure dysfunctional beliefs if the PM account of them is correct? One possible approach is suggested by the history of religious archetypes. According to Baring and Cashford (1991) the Great Mother had benign social consequences relative to the All Powerful Father in the Sky who, after going through various metamorphoses, eventually displaced Her in Western culture. The former, however, soon resurfaced in various guises, most prominently as Mary the Queen of Heaven in Catholicism, and is once more tempering ill effects of the Father. Perhaps this indicates that one should fight fire with fire, archetype with archetype. That this could be a high risk strategy is suggested by other historical examples, especially the manner in which rival archetypes in Ireland have slugged it out down the centuries without ever reaching any permanent accommodation.

Luckily for psychiatrists they do not usually have to deal with such powerful entities as the Sky Father, and the archetypes embodied in their patients responsible for some 'disease' are often quite insubstantial. The influence of the Healer can sometimes be enough to displace them, as the widespread popularity of faith healing shows. Some doctors are good at tapping into this archetype and using it constructively, though few would admit to doing so particularly in the present climate of opinion which leaves them wide open to accusations of quackery.

On the whole it may be best to avoid direct power struggles between personality-like archetypes of this sort even though this has always been an important part of the armoury of would-be therapists in every culture known to us. There is a limited place, perhaps, for trying to bring to life any beneficent archetype lacking in a patient. Many emotionally deprived people, for instance, lack the Nurturing Mother (among other figures) but the potential for bringing Her alive, especially in a group setting, is always there and can be used by the skilled or lucky doctor.

The best approach of all, when the psyche goes astray, may well be to invoke the assistance of the brain on which, after all, the psyche is largely dependent. Those parallel cognitive channels should be able to whittle away at any over-mighty archetype and cut it down to size. But how to assist them? In a sense we have come full circle since the obvious first step is to weaken the grip of the belief on the parallel channels which is what probably occurs when states of transmarginal inhibition are induced. Then the belief itself has to be shown up as simply one among several equally valid alternatives; i.e. the methods of cognitive therapy must be deployed. Maybe it was a mistake earlier on to say that cognitive therapy should remain divorced from the techniques of witch-doctors! The principles behind what they do could well be applied in our culture for ethical treatment, though so far they have been used mainly by those promoting religious movements of dubious worth. Of course, the setting in which treatment is undertaken can also aid or hinder the process of healing in a variety of subtle ways and merits separate discussion.

TREATMENT SETTINGS

There are a wide range of non-personal archetypes in addition to the personal ones that have been mentioned so far. An example that's particularly prominent at the moment is the Unstoppable Plague which complicates the lives of those trying to deal with AIDS. There are of course excellent rational grounds for fearing AIDS, but hardly for the degree of apprehensive emotion inspired by it. Even in Africa it causes on average fewer deaths than malaria, and in most developed countries presents almost identical risks and problems to Hepatitis B, quite a low-profile disease, although Hepatitis kills faster than AIDS. For a variety of reasons, the archetype quickly got attached to AIDS and has ever since loomed large, both as help and hindrance, in its management.

Two benign ideas that seem to be racial archetypes are the Sanctuary and the Healing Shrine. The Victorians were on the whole good at using archetypes to bolster their own purposes, and extended the Sanctuary into the Asylum for the treatment of mental disorders. In fact they overextended it which resulted in the backlash that we are still living through. Nevertheless, the idea of the Sanctuary has survived fairly intact, though somewhat weakened. The Healing Shrine has never lost its power. Witness the continuing appeal of Lourdes and similar places to the most unlikely people.

Both ideas got attached to hospitals where, at times, they probably did far more harm than good. It's extremely hard to account on any rational grounds, for instance, for the popularity of maternity hospitals (called lying-in hospitals) during the pre-antiseptic era. Mortality in these institutions due to sepsis following childbirth was often around 20 per cent (the 'natural' mortality due to childbirth being about 2 per cent). Only very powerful beliefs could have got women to go on dying in them in such numbers for nearly two centuries, whatever the additional social or other incentives. This power also has a potential for therapeutic benefit if harnessed in the right way. The Healing Shrine has all the potential value of the personal Healer for treating psychic disorders or disorders with a psychic component. Its drawbacks are of a longer-term, institutional sort compared to those of the Healer and are perhaps more easily monitored and controlled as long as there is an awareness of the need for keeping a regular eye on them.

Shrines are, however, places a little withdrawn from the community, served by acolytes who often wear distinctive clothes and usually speak little except to utter words of ritual or arcane mystery. This is a pretty good description of general hospitals as seen from a patient's point of view, but of course psychiatric services are trying to divest themselves of this image as fast as possible, while a whole range of social movements (from TV programmes like *Cardiac Arrest* to the Citizen's Charter) do their best to undermine it everywhere. It is healthy enough to debunk the archetype, given the lack of previous effective monitoring of drawbacks, but does tend to throw out the baby with the bathwater. As far as psychiatric services are concerned, the destruction of the Shrine is perhaps no bad thing in relation to treating primarily somatic disorders like schizophrenia or many depressions, but it removes a powerful weapon against those conditions that are actually psychic.

What seems to have happened in practice is that the weapon has not been so much removed as displaced from official psychiatric services to centres for holistic therapies and the like. The trouble with this is that the latter organisations escape monitoring just at a time when a very necessary appreciation of its importance is becoming widespread in the official services. Maybe there is still a place for shrines in the NHS psychiatric services. They have survived to date in a few specialist centres taking 'tertiary' referrals from local psychiatric services, but most such centres are in London and under threat from the new financial arrangements.

Another factor that needs to be taken into account in designing treatment settings is the quasi-infectious nature of the 'epidemic' psychic conditions. Patients are often apprehensive about being admitted to psychiatric units for fear that it will make them worse, meaning by this a fear that mental illness may be catching. When they ask questions about it they are generally told, if not in so many words, 'Of course not. Don't be so silly'. It's quite true that the serious brain illnesses like manic-depressive disorder and schizophrenia are certainly not catching, but unfortunately dysfunctional beliefs and behaviour patterns are only too transmissable. Psychiatrists generally do not like to think about this any more than the doctors attending lying-in hospitals liked to think about the consequences of their procedures. Nurses are often more realistic about facing up to the problem as it colours their whole working lives every day.

Particularly striking examples of behaviour transmission can be seen in services under strain when the normal, mostly unconscious, containment mechanisms break down. For instance, one service was in the process of transferring itself from a mental hospital to a district general hospital unit in a phased way when the first of Mrs Thatcher's restrictions on health service expenditure was promulgated. Incidentally, she herself clearly incarnated an archetype; some have suggested an aspect of the Great Mother but it's likely to have been a far more parochial one (the peculiarly English figure of Nanny Who Knows Best is a plausible candidate, though there were sometimes tinges of the Red Queen from Alice in Wonderland). Be this as it may, the service in question found itself, as a result of the cutbacks, restricted to half the planned number of beds for nearly three years. Staff coped, patient turnover increased, efficiency indicators (had there been such things at the time) must have rocketed. But some 24 in-patients killed themselves whereas the maximum expected number over the same period would have been 12. These were not people who ended their lives because they had been discharged too soon, but patients under active treatment who were getting more staff attention than they would have had under normal circumstances. Nor was what happened due to lack of staff vigilance or the like as efforts to prevent in-patient suicides were redoubled as soon as the epidemic became apparent. It was due to transmission of a behaviour that was facilitated in some ill-understood way by the financial and service pressures on the unit.

Clearly, it's important to design services in such a way that they don't transmit 'illness' of this sort. Obvious candidates for sceptical enquiry in this connection are the various community advisory services that have sprung up for problems with a psychic component, which don't actually offer curative treatment but do offer 'support' and 'counselling'. It's a commonplace, for instance, that the number of drug addicts in a town will appear to increase dramatically when an 'adequate' drugs advisory service is opened. This phenomenon is usually attributed to bringing hidden problems to light and, to a lesser extent, to attracting cases into the town from less-well-served areas.

Uncovering and concentrating cases may explain the entire apparent increase in disease incidence but it is instructive, though perhaps a little over-dramatic, to consider that similar explanations could have been given to acccount for the infamous water pump in London that was found to be spreading cholera in Victorian times; perhaps it just worsened or brought to light a cholera that was there anyway, or maybe it had some property which attracted cholera away from neighbouring pumps. It's not that safe to assume, in the absence of adequate epidemiological research, that a service will necessarily produce the effect intended. The expertise that exists concerning the epidemiology of infectious diseases could, and perhaps should, be extended in a rigorous way to the psychic illnesses. The crucial thing to remember is that a service which does not offer effective cures for its customers at the very least lays itself open to the risk of perpetuating some illnesses and spreading others that have an infective or quasi-infective basis.

Consideration must also be given to the likelihood that staff running a service are not immune to the epidemic psychic illnesses, not in the sense of themselves being liable to develop overt disease though occasionally this happens, but rather in getting infected by dysfunctional belief and becoming carriers of illness. There seems little doubt that Da Costa and like-minded colleagues helped to spread effort syndrome, and numerous contemporary examples of what is probably the same phenomenon could be cited. I won't try citing them because to do so would cause grave offence to some people and there is always the possibility of being wrong in some cases; reasonable certainty is only available to hindsight or to rigorous epidemiology. All the same, staff need to build up immunity to infectious beliefs, both those prevalent in the community and those to which specialists are prone. This can only be done by concentrating them in units and professional groupings containing a strong sceptical, academic component. The present fad for decentralising anything that can be decentralised and making academics 'accountable' is a recipe for disaster in relation to the psychic illnesses. Even in relation to somatic illness, it is not very sensible as a certain critical mass of professionals is needed simply to provide the range of skills and facilities required for optimum treatment. Together with properly evaluated preventive measures (vaccination and the like), maintaining chronic patients for whom there is no cure is about the only sensible goal for care in the community; but only after one has made absolutely sure that it's not simply a second best which saves everyone the bother of trying to find a proper answer.

Enough has been said to allow one to specify the outlines of a good PM paradigm psychic treatment service. It would not be very like most current services, and even less like the goal that we are encouraged to aim for under the banner of 'Care in the Community'. First of all, it would be quite highly centralized; acolytes might go out from it to spread the word and visit the sick, but they would soon return for peer group support and psychic decontamination. People working for it might actually *wear uniforms* or at least distinctive clothing of some sort. They would not be frowned upon for using professional language that outsiders would need to make an effort to understand. The architecture of the service base would be distinctive in some way. Sargant's own service at St Thomas's Hospital was a good example of the sort of thing that is required. Out-patients were seen in small, austere cells in the basement of the hospital. They had to be approached through gloomy corridors lined with rumbling water pipes, rather as a postulant might have had to approach the shrine of Mithras. In-patients were housed in a large penthouse on top of an old general hospital; one reached it in an airy cage of a lift which ascended creakingly through various nether regions before emerging in the light.

So far, we've given a recipe for an obscurantist, precious in the worst sense, service that could quickly go right off the rails. The vital thing to get right would be its internal structure. There would be resemblances to a religious community, so lessons could be learned from the organisation of monasteries and convents which, after all, managed to keep scholarship, education and some medical services going through a millennium of the most adverse social circumstances imaginable. An absolute essential would be to have within the organisation a strong, independent, academic unit in a position to evaluate and criticise all that was done, but also with some managerial powers. In addition, of course, the service would have to be protected somehow from the short-term fads of its paymasters. Utopias are more easily envisaged than constructed!

The Healing Shrine on its own is insufficient; it must be supplemented by the Sanctuary for those in need of short-term relief or long-term asylum. The present design for the Sanctuary is to put people in small privatised nursing homes or ersatz family units termed 'group homes'. The archetype is almost unrecognisable in this scheme which one can safely predict will come to grief. To be sure, the Home is itself a powerful and beneficent archetype, but not one that lends itself to artificial provision, least of all for those who have already proved unable to keep their own homes. Apart from anything else, it is not possible to adequately supervise or ensure a uniform standard of care in such a multiplicity of small units. Scandals of neglect or maltreatment will surely ensue. The Victorian conception of the Sanctuary was far more apt, at least in its origins. What went wrong as it developed was that it first got confused with the notion of the workhouse ('Industrial Therapy' remained popular right up to the recent era of high unemployment), and then with the social dumping ground or waste bin for misfits and nuisances. The resultant asylums had become quite horrific by the 1930s or 1940s; subsequent reforms came too late to redeem them.

A modern Sanctuary might be a bit like an up-market holiday camp; Center Parcs, for instance. Villas scattered through parkland with a phantasmagorical social and recreational area in the middle. To those who objected to the expense, one could point out that the weekly cost of a stay at Center Parcs, even in the high season, is about the same as keeping someone in a medium dependency nursing home while Butlins is less. Cultivating the holiday camp image too much would of course invite a backlash ('Why should I pay for all these idle so-and-sos to live in luxury while I have to go out to work'), but nevertheless a Sanctuary with such benign associations might escape the evils which quickly overcame the Victorian attempt to embody it.

CONCLUSIONS

Whatever else may be said about the PM set of ideas when applied in some detail to a field, they are not dull. In relation to medicine, they seem to illuminate some rather obscure corners in a constructive way. They suggest some wholly new treatments as well as new ways of increasing the effectiveness of old ones. They also seem to fit in better in some contexts than HE ideas with that often invoked, but rarely defined, sacred cow 'clinical experience'. Few psychiatrists believe deep down that the soma is all, though most pay lip service to the notion because of the prevailing intellectual climate. The PM paradigm offers a rational means of escape from what many feel to be a type of unwarranted intellectual imprisonment.

If these ideas turn out to be correct they will require quite major, but to some welcome, upheavals in the way that psychic treatment services are provided. Although it may be all right to treat the body as a commodity in the health service market, the idea is so ludicrously inappropriate in relation to the PM notion of the psyche that no compromise could be reached. What is happening at present is that psychic treatment services are being driven to an unregulated fringe where there is a risk that they will fester. Meanwhile, mainstream services are left in an unbalanced condition which is unsustainable in the long term because, to deal with the soma only leaving out the psyche, is a bit like hopping instead of walking. Perhaps paradoxically, these considerations suggest that there are strong economic arguments for funding very basic research into the nature of the psyche. Until we know more about it, we won't know how best to spend a large proportion of health service budgets.

REFERENCES

Baring, A. and Cashford, J. (1991) *The Myth of the Goddess*, BCA: London, New York.

Birtchnell, J. (1994) 'Battle for the Mind – a Physiology of Conversion and Brainwashing: William Sargant', *British Journal of Psychiatry* 164, 273–5.

Cooper, C.L. and Faragher, B.E. (1993) 'Psychosocial Stress and Breast Cancer: The Inter-relationship between Stress Events, Coping Strategies and Personality', *Psychological Medicine* 23, 653–62.

Da Costa, J.M. (1871) 'On Irritable Heart: A Clinical Study of a Form of Functional Cardiac Disorder and its Consequences', *Journal of the American Medical Society* 61, 17.

Dunbar, F. (1954) *Emotions and Bodily Changes* (4th edn), Columbia University Press: New York.

Hinckle, L.E. and Wolff, H.F. (1957) 'The Nature of Man's Adaptation to his Total Environment and the Relation of this to Illness', *Archives of Internal Medicine* 99, 442–60.

Ho, M-W. (1994) 'Towards an Indigenous Western Science: Causality in the Universe of Coherent Space-Time Structures', in *New Metaphysical Foundations of Modern Science*, W. Harman and J. Clark (eds), Institute of Noetic Sciences, California.

Hughes, J. (1991) *An Outline of Modern Psychiatry* (3rd edn), Wiley: Chichester.

Jung, C.G. (1939) 'On the Psychogenesis of Schizophrenia', in *Collected Works of C.G. Jung*, vol. 3 (1960 edn), Routledge & Kegan Paul: London.

Leigh, D. (1968) 'The Form Complete. The Present State of Psychosomatic Medicine', *Proceedings of the Royal Society of Medicine* 61, 375–84.

Morgagni, J.B. (1761) *The Seats and Causes of Disease* (transl. B. Alexander, 1769), Millar and Cadell: London.

Munich, R.L. (1993) 'Group Dynamics', in *Comprehensive Group Psychotherapy* (3rd edn), H.I. Kaplan and B.J. Sadock (eds), Williams and Wilkins: Baltimore.

Nunn, C.M.H. (1974) 'The Relationship between Physical Disease and Affective Disorder in Old People' (MD thesis, University of London).

O'Donnell, M. (1994) 'Anecdotal Evidence: Persecuted by Counsellors', *Healthcare Management*, April, 60.

Parry-Jones, B. (1991) 'Historical Terminology of Eating Disorders', *Psychological Medicine* 21, 21–8.

Roessler, R. and Greenfield, N.S. (1961) 'Incidence of Somatic Disease in Psychiatric Patients', *Psychosomatic Medicine* 23(5), 413–19.

Sargant, W. (1957) *Battle for the Mind*, William Heinemann: London.

Selye, H. (1950) *Stress*, Act Inc.: Montreal.

Tourenne, C.J. (1985) 'A Model of the Electric Field of the Brain at EEG and Microwave Frequencies', *Journal of Theoretical Biology* 116, 495–507.

Treasure, J. and Campbell I. (1994) 'The Case for Biology in the Aetiology of

Anorexia Nervosa', *Psychological Medicine* 24, 3–8.

Trethowan, W.H. (1988) 'Pain as a Psychiatric Symptom', in *Perspectives in Psychiatry*, P. Hall and P.D. Stonier (eds), Wiley: Chichester.

Wessely, S. (1990) 'Old Wine in New Bottles: Neurasthenia and ME', *Psychological Medicine* 20, 35–53.

Wood, G.C., Bentall, R.P., Gopfert, M., Dewey, M.E. and Edwards, R.H.T. (1994) 'The Differential Response of Chronic Fatigue, Neurotic and Muscular Dystrophy Patients to Experimental Psychological Stress', *Psycholological Medicine* 24, 357–64.

9 Towards a science of the soul?

It's a little unfair to the two paradigms that they have been set up as opponents; two straw men knocking each other about and scoring points whenever one does something that the other can't. They should in truth be allies. The relationship between them is analogous to that between Newtonian gravitational theory (for HE ideas) and General Relativity (for PM ones). General Relativity did not contradict Newton's laws so much as subsume and extend them. For many practical purposes, it is easier and just as satisfactory to stick with Newton; you only need Einstein to deal with extreme cases and to provide overall understanding. It took careful observation of rather rare and subtle phenomena to distinguish between the two physical theories when there was still doubt about which was more true. As far as the HE/PM distinction is concerned, only the most preliminary of observations have been made but, if later ones should confirm the PM approach, HE theories will nevertheless remain valid in their area of application; it will simply be a matter of having shown that what they cover, at present thought by some to be everything to do with the mind, is really a fenced-off subsection of a larger field.

Crick (the co-discoverer of the structure of DNA, who switched to working on problems to do with brain and mind a good many years ago) calls his version of the HE paradigm *The Astonishing Hypothesis*. It's tempting to comment that he must astonish easily. All the same, in relation to Cartesian dualism which held the field for so long, it is startling to propose as he does that there might be nothing to the mind but neural activity. It's also very restricting. Whole areas of study and thought, to say nothing of much folk psychology which can be referred to in a more flattering light as the accumulated self-knowledge of innumerable generations, must be abandoned or fitted into the strait-jacket of brain words. But this abstemiousness is in all likelihood *unnecessary*. 'All likelihood' can actually be defined as 500 to 1 at present! One is perfectly at liberty, on the PM view, to examine in the most narrowly classical scientific terms the reflexive patterns of activity in neural nets which underpin so much of mental life *and* consider, say, the reciprocal influences of archetypes and artistic sensibilities using a language that retains the advantages gained hitherto by people specialising in each field, but which is also enriched by the addition of quantum concepts.

A brief PM definition of the soul would have to identify it with the succession of Bose condensates in the brain. In principle there should even be the possibility of measuring its radiative field, weak though it is. But then all sorts of qualifications would have to be introduced. The Bose condensates are only demi-semi-independent of underlying classical neural activity which certainly makes the largest contribution to the content of soul on any quantitative basis. Condensates are also, to an extent, enmeshed with the world around them which includes other people and their condensates. Any dividing line put between the individual soul and its physical and social environment is bound to be sometimes arbitrary. There are unified, if often rather insubstantial, entities at various levels from family through nation and race, culminating presumably in a soul of the biosphere – the famous Gaia hypothesis.

There is a big problem with this concept in that the Bose condensates in any individual brain have been pictured as succeeding one another at a rate of around 10 per second. Does this mean that one must think, not of *the* soul of a person, but of a succession of souls being born and snuffed out at this rate? If not, how can continuity between successive condensates be envisaged? An austere person would no doubt say that the picture of a rapid succession of souls in any individual has to be accepted, but then someone like this would probably be stuck with the HE paradigm and so would not agree that there is a real problem. Reasons have already been found for thinking that intellectual abstemiousness may sometimes be a mistake so let us assume, for the sake of argument, that it would also be mistaken in this connection.

Continuity of a sort as far as the *content* of awareness (i.e. soul) is concerned is of course maintained by neural mechanisms such as attention. During sleep this is mostly lost so awareness flits about capriciously; all the same there is a sense of self still present in (probably) all dreams. Is there perhaps something about the self-model that provides continuity between successive Bose condensates, so linking them into one continuous soul? This suggestion has a certain appeal and is probably true as far as the classical activity underlying awareness of self is concerned. The self-model is almost always activated whenever the brain is conscious, so providing an awareness of a continuing self. In Chapter 4 the self was envisaged as the frame of a mirror in which awareness reflects the world. However, the self-model is only a mechanism or a range of mechanisms of some sort, and is on the other side of the dualistic divide from awareness itself, so this won't really do as an answer to the problem. If inclined to think it satisfactory, one has only to consider how continuity of soul can be conceived after a period of anaesthesia or coma or even very deep sleep. There ought to be a gap in these circumstances. The revived awareness should surely be regarded as a separate, new soul different from the one that preceded unconsciousness.

Perhaps all this is a category mistake, that bane of philosophical enquiry. Soul should not be conceived as a thing but as an abstraction in which case it is entirely satisfactory to think that other abstractions, such as the information content in a self-model, can provide continuity for it. Unfortunately, this won't do either. The essence of the PM perspective is that awareness is a thing that may, if one takes a Platonic view, have a greater degree of thingness than the body which supports it. Of course, the body, which seems to us so stable, in fact replaces almost all its constituent molecules every few months. Some parts of it, blood for instance, have an even faster turnover time of a matter of a few weeks. Maybe, to come full circle, the unchanging identity over time of the soul is as illusory as that of the body.

The fact that this argument is going round in circles probably indicates a lack of the right concepts for dealing with the continuity of anything over time. Awareness, and hence soul, is a quantum entity but quantum theory does not cope well with time; it can provide only hints but no definitive guidelines. One of the hints that was extracted towards the end of Chapter 3 was that uniqueness of shape might modify the likelihood that all possible pasts of a quantum object exist in superposition in such a way as to result in there being only one possible past for objects of unique shape (readers should remember that this *is* pure speculation). If there is anything to this idea one could argue that there would also be a unique aspect to the shape of any individual's Bose condensates dependent on the form of the quantum representation of his or her self-model. Just possibly this might provide a link between successive condensates allowing them to build over time a unique history that would have some of the characteristics of a single (four-dimensional (4D)) object. Maybe it is legitimate to talk of a PM soul possessing true continuity and not just the appearance of it, though only speculation is possible until the quantum theory of time becomes firmer than is the case at present.

There's an analogy to be made between music and this idea of soul: music consists of a series of individual notes, while soul is a series of qualia. Yet a particular piece of music may possess a quality that can only be described as 'personality' (see Rowell, 1993). Somehow a particular succession of vibrations in the air builds an individual character, recognisable by anyone with an ear for such things. The analogy can't be pressed very far as the links between notes are made in someone's mind while those between qualia, if they occur at all, are due to the properties of space-time; but it does illustrate a point about how fleeting entities may build something much more enduring.

There are innumerable 'buts' and 'what ifs?' that can be raised around this concept. For instance, what if someone's self-model is badly damaged by injury or illness; does this mean his previous soul dies in some sense and he gets a new one? Well maybe sometimes yes, despite the earlier pooh-poohing of the idea that a person might get a new soul after a good sleep, provided that the new self-model shape is sufficiently different from the old one. After anaesthaesia, or the like, the shape of the self-model is unaltered so continuity of soul is unaffected by that sort of hiatus, but the situation may be very different after severe head injury, for example. It's only too common for the spouse of a brain-damaged person, or the parents of an incorrigible drug addict, to say that the person has become a total stranger, 'just not the man I married', or 'not the son I knew'. This is normally taken as a figure of speech, but perhaps it can be the literal truth.

Whatever its legitimacy, the notion that souls might be 4D quantum objects has a certain appeal and is worth playing with a little more. One straightforward implication is that the 'signature' of any individual soul should in principle be observable by looking at the topological characteristics of microwave radiation relating to the person's self-model. If something can be observed, it can be studied using ordinary scientific methods.

At the opposite end of the philosophical spectrum, the idea has implications for how one should regard the value of awareness, previously touched on in Chapter 7, where it was speculated that our sort of consciousness might be regarded as adding to the variety and beauty of the universe. If awareness possesses a unique continuity, it must be thought of as doing something much more definite; namely, creating a definite past for a universe in which, without awareness, all possible pasts would coexist in what might be considered a chaotic jumble. People have often wondered whether consciousness might in some sense create its own present and we have to agree here that there is a limited sense in which this is true. It does make a small contribution to defining the present, though mostly its present is created for it by external circumstances and classical brain activity. Thinking that it might in a strong sense 'fix' the past is not so familiar, though the idea has a respectable pedigree (Davies, 1986). All the same, it's a clear implication of the view of soul that has been reached here. Stapp (1994) has shown mathematically that slight, plausible modifications of standard quantum theory result in backward causation being something that is bound to happen. He wanted to explain some strange experimental results. It seems that people's later wishes can affect random events that happened months previously and were recorded but never seen by anyone until after the wishes had been made. This, if true, is not quite the same phenomenon as is involved in the proposal made here that awareness eliminates all but one past from the superposition of past events that occurs in its absence, but the backward causation involved may be similar.

This line of thought also requires that a degree of 4D unity must be allowed to what have been termed 'archetypes'. Although they are spatially more diffused (occupying separate brains instead of separate areas within a single brain), they have a similar enduring continuity of shape to that envisaged for the souls of individuals. These entities have affinities with what Dawkins (1976) has called 'memes' to resonate with genes. Memes are ideas, beliefs, etc. that use brains and other information stores to reproduce themselves just as genes use bodies. They tend to behave like bacteria or viruses in that some can help their hosts while others spread like a plague leaving trails of damage in their wake. As in the case of the 'selfish gene', their *raison d'être* is their own survival and whether they harm or help the bodies that give them life is determined entirely by whether doing so aids their own spread.

There are differences between archetypes and memes. Archetypes are embodied only in brains, though they can be transmitted from brain to brain via books, computers or whatever, whereas memes are more abstract and are fully themselves even when occupying a printed page rather than someone's cortex. Memes are also simpler in structure as a rule, and rarely personal. Nevertheless, meme theory must apply to some extent to archetypes which have to be envisaged as quasi-biological entities, dependent on the brains that give them existence but following their own laws as they flourish and decay. Their beneficence or otherwise in relation to us as individuals is determined only by which qualities will aid their own survival in a world of competing archetypes. To envisage the existence of supra-personal souls like these has obvious implications for almost every field of study. In fact there are probably no areas of human thought or activity which would be unaffected by such entities. Even quite superficial consequences would require volumes to explore, so better not to start here!

This view of both personal and archetypal 'soul' implies that its principal attribute other than awareness must be memory. A soul *is* a unique history in one guise or another. In the Introduction it was claimed that much awareness might be forgotten or inherently unrememberable and that this makes for all sorts of difficulties when it comes to thinking about consciousness. This claim may have been just as misleading as the slightly later one (beginning of Chapter 1) that you can't have awareness without a brain to have it in. It may well be a consequence of the PM outlook that awareness is *always* remembered in the sense of being imprinted on the structure of space-time. Of course, this does not mean that every past awareness will in practice be recallable in the sense of being capable of reproduction at will by classical neural activity in our brains, but it probably does mean that all awareness that has ever occurred can in principle be remembered. This is nice, if true, in that it removes most of a major obstacle to getting to grips with consciousness. It's not so nice in that there is much in the past which might be better consigned to oblivion.

The speculation opens up a potential field of enquiry even wider than that implicit in the suggestion that archetypes may exist as quasi-biological entities. A possibility that memories of past lives might sometimes be veridical, as New Age enthusiasts so often claim, is among the most obvious implications, though it would not entail a belief in reincarnation. Maybe people can get access to stray memories imprinted on the fabric of the universe that are not part of their own personal histories, but seem personal in the absence of any other referents.

So many extensive vistas open out from the PM approach to awareness that one cannot help but wish it might be true. Truth, however, is important while wishful thinking isn't. Getting at truth in this context needs painstaking scientific study. A lot more such work will have to be done before anyone can be reasonably certain that the HE view can't account for all the phenomena of consciousness. The balance of probabilities does favour PM theories, but that's not enough to satisfy most of us.

REFERENCES

Davies, P. (1986) 'Time Asymmetry and Quantum Mechanics', in *The Nature of Time*, R. Flood and M. Lockwood (eds), Basil Blackwell: Oxford.

Dawkins, R. (1976) *The Selfish Gene*, Oxford University Press.

Rowell, L. (1993) 'Music as Process', in *Time and Process*, J.T. Fraser and

L. Rowell (eds), International Universities Press.
Stapp, H.P. (1994) 'Theoretical Model of a Purported Empirical Violation of the Predictions of Quantum Theory', *Physics Review A.* 50(1), 18–22.

Glossary

Abreaction The technique of getting someone to relive a traumatic past experience, or the process of reliving such an experience.

Agoraphobia Literally fear of the market-place. Sufferers tend to experience acute anxiety if they leave home, travel on buses, visit a supermarket, etc.

Archetype A recurrent theme in people's imagination or awareness. Used by Jung to refer to themes shared by the entire human race, but in this book as a term for trends in awareness in smaller groups as well as those to be found in the race as a whole.

ATP Adenosine triphosphate. A chemical whose breakdown (to the diphosphate) provides the principal, immediate source of energy for cellular activities.

Awareness Used here as a synonym for 'consciousness': the state of being aware which is available to introspection.

Axon The most substantial and longest process(es) belonging to a nerve cell. Lesser processes are called 'dendrites'.

Behaviourism The school of psychology which held that animals (and people) should be regarded as 'black boxes' for scientific purposes. Responses to stimuli should be studied, it was said, but there's no point in thinking about what might be going on between stimulus and response.

Binding problem The problem of how it is that activity in different parts of the brain combines to give a unified experience.

Bose–Einstein condensate A state of profound harmony between quantum particles in their aspects as waves which results in their losing individual identity and becoming a unity.

Boson Any sub-atomic particle possessing integral (i.e. 0, 1 or 2) spin.

Brain stem The part of the brain linking spinal chord to cerebral hemispheres.

Cartesian dualism The proposition, due to the philosopher Descartes, that body and soul are largely independent of one another but are weakly linked in a specific part of the brain.

Cerebellum A part of the brain, situated at the rear below the cerebral hemispheres, which is thought to aid the control of movement and may also have other functions.

(Cerebral) cortex The layer of nerve cells which covers the surface of the cerebral hemispheres.

Cerebral hemispheres These form the main bulk of nervous tissue in humans comprising, as they do, the part of the brain above the level of the thalamus. Although interconnected, they are clearly divided into two, one on the right and the other on the left. Anatomists have defined various subdivisions of each hemisphere, at the coarsest level into frontal, parietal, temporal and occipital lobes.

Classical Used here to refer to any scientific theory or explanation which does *not* make use of quantum concepts.

Cochlea The organ in the inner ear which converts sound vibrations into nerve impulses.

Cognitive To do with knowing: the term relates more to the intellectual than the emotional aspects of comprehension. Cognitive psychology studies people's habitual ways of construing their worlds, in addition to how perception translates into knowledge of the environment.

Coherence The occurrence of frequency matching and synchronisation of two or more wave-forms that may previously have been independent. It is used in connection with both ordinary wave-forms, such as EEG ones, and quantum, Schrodinger waves.

Depolarisation wave Used here to refer to a reduction in the voltage across a nerve cell membrane that spreads in a wave-like manner over the cell to its furthest ramifications.

Dipole Used here to refer to molecules which have an opposite electrical charge at either end.

Dopamine One of the monoamine neurotransmitters.

Dualism A term used here to refer to the view that mind and brain are distinguishable.

EEG (electro-encephalogram or -ography) The record of, and/or the technique of recording, the electrical activity of the brain. Recordings are usually made from electrodes placed on the scalp, but in exceptional circumstances electrodes may touch the brain.

Electrical potential A voltage: used here mainly to refer to a voltage difference between one side of a cell membrane and the other.

Epidemiology The study of the distribution and spread of diseases.

Epiphenomenon An irrelevant associate of something, or an unimportant and unefficacious secondary result of something, e.g. the froth on a breaking wave.

Epistemology The study of the basis of knowledge.

Evoked potential Refers to a voltage change detected by EEG consequent on an external input to the brain, usually a sensory stimulus of some sort.

Frontal lobe The most anterior part of a cerebral hemisphere. Its functions are complex and have to do with attention, motivation, fine emotional discriminations, etc.

Gauge theory A physical theory which shows how the fundamental forces can be explained on a common basis and, in so doing, accounts for the range of observed sub-atomic particles. So far, only three of the four forces have been successfully included; gravity remains elusive.

Global workspace A concept drawn from computer design. A global workspace takes the output from one or a few of a range of competing processors and distributes it, with or without modification, to all the processors.

Goldstone boson A quantum particle without mass which, it is hypothesised, can be generated by breaking symmetry of activity in neural nets.

Graviton The (hypothetical) quantum particle of gravity.

GTP Guanosine triphosphate. An analogue of ATP which also provides an energy source for cells. GTP is associated with microtubules; it appears to help stabilise their ends as they grow.

HE Paradigm The group of theories which share as a basic premise the notion that consciousness emerges from classical interactions between nerve cells. 'HE' refers to Hofstadter and Edelman; two well-known proponents of this idea.

Hippocampus A part of the limbic system which is situated in the temporal lobe. They (there is one on each side) are thought to have a special role in transforming short-term into permanent memory.

Hz (or hertz) A unit of frequency. 1 Hz = 1 cycle per second.

Laser light A beam of photons of exactly the same frequency and precisely in phase. It is produced by the process of lasing which involves triggering excited molecules to release their energy in concert.

Limbic system An important system of nerve cells and fibre tracts linking thalami and cerebral hemispheres on either side. It plays a part in emotions, particularly flight/fight ones, and memory.

Locus coerulus Literally, the blue place: a small group of nerve cells in the upper part of the brain stem.

MEG (Magneto-encephalogram or -ography) The record of, and/or the technique of recording, the brain's magnetic fields.

Microtubule A cylindrical structure inside a cell, made of protein components called tubulin. Microtubules ramify throughout all cells, including nerve cells. They are sometimes regarded as the cell's 'skeleton', but are known to be dynamic structures that play an essential part in cell movement and cell division; they are suspected of having other roles, too.

Msec (or millesecond) A unit of time. 1 msec. =.001 seconds.

Neural network A group of neurones which are interconnected in such a way that only a few intermediate steps are required to transmit information between the most widely separated of the cells. The term also refers to computer simulations of this situation.

Neurone Means the same as 'nerve cell'.

Neurotransmitter Any chemical released by a nerve cell which influences other nerve cells by binding to receptors in the cell surface membrane. Most neurones have autoreceptors for their own neurotransmitter(s) which can modulate the amount released or produced.

Neutron star A collapsed star made of degenerate matter (neutronium). They are typically twice as heavy as our sun, but only 15 miles in diameter.

Occipital lobe The part of a cerebral hemisphere underlying the back of the head. Its cortex is used for vision.

Olfactory bulb The part of the brain from which nerve fibres originate that end in the lining of the nose. It subserves the sense of smell.

Organic Used here to mean that something pertains to the physical or somatic rather than the mental or psychic.

Paradigm A pattern of thought. Used here in the Kuhnian manner to mean a group of scientific theories sharing common characteristics.

Parietal lobe The upper-middle part of a cerebral hemisphere. Two of its functions have to do with appreciating touch sensations and controlling movements.

Phonon The quantum particle corresponding to the energy of mechanical vibration.

Photon The quantum particle of electro-magnetic vibrational energy, which includes light.

PM Paradigm The group of theories which hold that consciousness can be fully understood only through using some of the concepts of quantum theory. 'PM' refers to Penrose and Marshall, who have proposed ideas of this type.

Psyche The mental aspect of a person. At one time regarded as equivalent to spirit or soul, the term has become drained of meaning as a materialist view of mind has spread.

Psychosomatic Referring to the importance of both mental (psychic) and bodily (somatic) factors in relation to something, usually disease.

q.e.d. The traditional ending for a mathematical proof. Stands for: quod erat demonstrandum. Means: it's been proved or, literally, which was to be demonstrated.

Quale (pl. qualia) A perceptual quality such as 'blueness': but used in this book in a more general sense to refer to the content of consciousness at any given moment.

Quantum Used as a noun, this is the smallest quantity of anything that can exist. The concept was first employed in connection with energy but also, it is thought, applies to electric charge, angular momentum, length, time, gravity. A quantum of light is a photon; a quantum of electricity an electron. Used as an adjective, it is commonly an abbreviation for 'quantum theoretical'.

Quantum object Anything which can be accurately described only in terms of quantum theory.

Receptor Used here to refer to the structures in nerve cell surface membranes which are the chemical 'locks' for which neurotransmitters are the 'keys'.

Relative state formulation Otherwise known as the 'many worlds' hypothesis; a variant is called the 'many biographies' hypothesis. A reformulation of quantum mechanics due to Everett which is attractive to theoreticians as it does away with the awkward conceptual problems surrounding the idea of wave function collapse. Many consider, however, that the cure is worse than the disease!

REM sleep The phase of sleep characterised by rapid eye movements and faster EEG activity.

Reticular activating system A network of nerve cells in the core of the brain stem.

Schizophrenia A serious psychiatric illness characterised by the experience of hallucinations and delusions, emotional upsets and often by loss of qualities such as drive and capacity to feel deeply.

Serotonin One of the monoamine neurotransmitters: also known as 5–hydroxytryptamine.

Slow wave sleep The phase of sleep characterised by high amplitude, slow EEG activity.

Solipsism The belief that only one's own consciousness is knowable: other people might be unconscious zombies or the outside world as a whole could be a figment of one's imagination.

Soliton (Davydov soliton) Solitary waves that can appear in a variety of circumstances and carry energy. They can also be regarded as quantum particles corresponding to the energy of elastic deformation.

Soma The body; especially when considered in relation to the psyche.

Somatosensory Relating to bodily sensation: e.g. relating to touch as opposed to vision.

Spin The quantum property of 'spin' is sometimes pictured as analogous to angular momentum, such as that possessed by a spinning cricket ball. However, this analogy is misleading as a quantum particle can possess 'spin' in several different directions at the same time. I doubt if anyone can form an accurate picture of the phenomenon except in mathematical terms.

Strange attractor A mathematical concept used in chaos theory. It is the 'centre' of a pattern of chaotic activity.

Superposition The quantum state in which alternative potential realities can coexist.

Synapse A structure formed by a terminal branch of one nerve cell and the adjacent surface of another cell.

Syndrome A pattern of circumstances. In relation to disease, a group of symptoms and/or signs of illness that commonly occur together.

Temporal lobe The lower-middle part of a cerebral hemisphere. Its functions are complex and poorly understood.

Temporal lobe epilepsy A form of epilepsy originating in a temporal lobe. Sufferers often go blank for a short while or experience a stereotyped sensation of some sort, but may not have convulsions.

Thalamus Two important groups of nerve cells (one on each side) situated at the top of the brain stem. Each contains a number of subsidiary nerve cell groups, some of which have sensory functions while others have roles in emotion and memory.

Tomography The technique of producing cross-sectional images by integrating information about direction and intensity provided by particles (or waves) that have traversed or originated from a body.

Topology The branch of mathematics dealing with shape.

Transcendental meditation A technique claimed to induce inner peace, harmony and relaxation through the concentration of attention on some thought or object suggested by an instructor.

Transmarginal inhibition A state of altered brain function, first described by Pavlov, which manifests itself in changes in conditioned reflexes. It can be caused by severe stress and probably by repetitive, rhythmic stimulation.

Tubulin A generic name for the group of proteins that form the structure of microtubules – other proteins often adhere to this structure. There are at least twenty different types, though any individual microtubule contains only a few types arranged regularly in a quasi-crystalline pattern (usually a skewed hexagonal lattice).

Veridical Corresponding with reality.

Wave function (or Schrodinger wave function) The mathematical expression of quantum theory developed by Schrodinger. The wave function consists of probability amplitudes which represent every possibility that a quantum object is capable of manifesting.

Wave function collapse The event which transforms the cloud of potentialities in a Schrodinger wave function into a single actuality. The mathematical operation corresponding to it is to square the probability amplitudes, so converting the imaginary numbers that partially describe these amplitudes into real ones. What this could mean in physical terms is the subject of much debate.

Weak nuclear force One of the four fundamental forces known to physicists. The others are the strong nuclear force, electro-magnetism and gravity.

Name index

Subject index

abreaction 56, 128, 135, 155
agoraphobia 155; *see also* 'anxiety'
AIDS 140
allergy to the twentieth century 129
alpha rhythm: *see* EEG
anaesthesia 93, 151; hysterical 21
anaesthetics 6–7, 29, 78
animal consciousness 109–12
ant fugue 62–3
ants, white 111
anxiety 125, 130–1
archetypes 118, 131–3, 137, 139–41,
    142, 149, 152–3, 155
artificial intelligence 63; *see also* Tur-
    ing test
artists 106, 118–19
astrocytes 8
asylum 140, 144–5
ATP 13, 17, 71, 155
attention 13, 27, 34, 36, 95, 99–100,
    101 114, 149
awareness, and Bose condensates 70–
    6; conditions for occurrence of 6,
    27, 38–9, 121; definition of 1;
    efficaciousness of 65, 86, 99, 110,
    112–13; fragmentation of 20–3, 25–
    7, 78, 102; functions of 99, 112–17,
    151–2; information content of 14–
    15; mirror analogy 5, 76; theories of
    59–76; timing of 37–41, 42, 72–3, 74

backward causation 56, 152
beauty 105–7, 118
belief 75–6, 136–7, 138–9, 141–2
binding problem 9–10, 35, 42, 70, 77,
    155
blindsight 26–7
Bose–Einstein condensates 28, 53–4,
    122, 155; relationship of to con-
    sciousness 70–6, 112–13; topology
    of 17, 56, 73, 76, 77, 107, 118, 150
bosons 53

brain, anatomy 9–11; clocks 32–4;
    electrical activity 11–12, 19, 24;
    imaging techniques 23, 98, 134;
    injury to 6, 24–7, 102, 129, 151;
    purpose of 14, 117–19; stem 10–11,
    27, 78, 100, 155; words 97–8, 105,
    125, 136

Capgras syndrome 22–3
cerebellum 4, 156
cerebral cortex: *see* cortex
chaotic nervous activity 16, 68–9, 96
Chinese room argument 65, 103
chronic fatigue syndromes: *see* effort
    syndrome and myalgic encephalo-
    myelitis
cognition 11, 18, 24, 57, 61, 104, 118,
    138, 156
cognitive impairment 125
cognitive therapy 136, 140
coherence studies: *see* EEG,
    correlated activity
complex numbers 45–6
condensates: *see* Bose–Einstein con-
    densates
consciousness: *see* awareness
contingent negative variation: *see*
    expectancy wave
corpus callosum 25
correlated EEG activity: *see* EEG
cortex 9–10, 27, 29, 110; mirror
    analogy 10, 29
counsellors 132–3, 142
cures 122–3, 133–40
cytoskeleton: *see* microtubules

Davydov soliton: *see* soliton
decision-making 36, 67, 69, 85, 97
delirium 22
depersonalisation/derealisation 127–8
depolarisation waves 12, 17, 28, 33,
    98, 156